AF816884

Audit, Service Evaluation and Research in Health and Social Care

Audit, Service Evaluation and Research in Health and Social Care

Getting started in project work

Helen Aveyard, Ginny Mounce and Kathleen Greenway

McGraw Hill
Open University Press

Open University Press
McGraw Hill
Unit 4
Foundation Park
Roxborough Way
Maidenhead
SL6 3UD

email: emea_uk_ireland@mheducation.com
world wide web: www.mheducation.co.uk

Copyright © Open International Publishing Limited, 2026

All rights reserved. Except for the quotation of short passages for the purposes of criticism and review, no part of this publication may be reproduced, stored in a retrieval system, or transmitted, in any form or by any means, electronic, mechanical, photocopying, recording or otherwise, without the prior written permission of the publisher or a licence from the Copyright Licensing Agency Limited. Details of such licences (for reprographic reproduction) may be obtained from the Copyright Licensing Agency Ltd of Saffron House, 6–10 Kirby Street, London EC1N 8TS.

Executive Editor: Hannah Church
Editorial Assistant: Molly Overend
Content Product Manager: Graham Jones

A catalogue record of this book is available from the British Library

ISBN-13: 9780335253500
ISBN-10: 0335253504
eISBN-13: 9780335253517

Typeset by Transforma Pvt. Ltd., Chennai, India

Fictitious names of companies, products, people, characters and/or data that may be used herein (in case studies or in examples) are not intended to represent any real individual, company, product or event.

010289 ACL 2026

Praise for this book

"Excellent for qualified and student healthcare professionals, this book provides a step-by-step guide through a variety of research projects. The authors' clear and thorough explanations of research terminology and procedures, make research concepts accessible and easy to navigate. The book covers all key research processes from deciding on a question to the dissemination of findings. The text is clearly laid out and supported with a variety of helpful worked examples. Overall, a highly suitable book for anyone embarking on a healthcare research project."

Philippa Beaumont, PGDip, BSc, FHEA,
Senior Lecturer in Physiotherapy, University of Winchester, UK.

"Audit, Service Evaluation and Research in Health and Social Care is a wonderful overview and a great starter text that will help undergraduate and postgraduate students gain confidence in using research skills to solve real problems by encouraging practical application from the outset. This book is easy to read with a logical progression through the stages of inquiry and problem-solving. Clear definitions and distinctions of terms demonstrate to the reader that starting small can be exciting and make a difference to patient outcomes and safety. The inclusion of equity, diversity and inclusivity as well as community engagement and involvement (PPI) is important and welcome."

Dr Amelia Swift, Reader in Health Professional Education,
University of Birmingham, UK.

"This book offers a clearly articulated exploration of audits, service evaluations, and small-scale research in health and social care practice. It presents complex concepts with precision and thoughtful organisation. The practical tools it provides help nurses and health and social care practitioners carry out clinical audits and service evaluations, building confidence in using evidence and applying it meaningfully in clinical settings. It is a highly valuable resource for nursing, health and social care students, educators, and practitioners committed to advancing evidence based care."

Dr Sabina Gerrard, Senior Lecturer, School of Nursing & Midwifery,
University of Central Lancashire, UK.

"This book is a welcome guide for anyone involved in audit, service evaluation or project work across health and social care. It is particularly valuable for trainee and advancing practitioners, for whom these activities are a core part of their identity. The authors bring together clear, practical advice in one accessible resource that helps practitioners build confidence and make real improvements in their services, contributing to excellent outcomes for patients and populations through the transformation of services."

Vicky MacArthur, Senior Lecturer in Advanced Clinical Practice, University of Cumbria, UK.

"This is an excellent resource for anyone beginning their research journey, particularly those undertaking smaller scale projects. It provides a contemporary, step-by-step guide that is clear, accessible and thoughtfully structured. The authors demystify key terminology, provide practical considerations and give timely guidance on the ethical use of AI. Real world examples vividly illustrate the distinctions and value of audit, service evaluation and research. I highly recommend this book as a reliable companion throughout the process, or for anyone seeking to understand these important differences."

Gemma Breitschadel, Senior Lecturer (Nursing Apprenticeship), University College Birmingham, UK.

"This book is an invaluable guide for students undertaking research, audits or service evaluations. It clearly explains how "small scale projects provide essential research training" and shows how such work strengthens evidence based practice. By breaking down each stage from forming a focused question to ethical approval, data collection and analysis the text offers practical, confidence building support. Its emphasis on real world examples, rigorous methods and achievable project design makes it an empowering companion for learners who want to improve services, deepen understanding and contribute meaningfully to patient care."

Professor Ian Jones RN, PhD, Professor of Cardiovascular Nursing, Liverpool John Moores University, UK.

Contents

Introduction

As you are reading this book, you are probably about to embark on a research journey – be that an audit, service evaluation or research project. Whether you are studying for an undergraduate, master's or doctoral award, this book provides a guide to undertaking a small-scale study. We identify the key concepts that are relevant to small-scale projects and signpost you to other resources for information that is beyond the scope of this book. We hope you find this a useful companion to your studies.

Research provides the evidence to inform patient or client care. It is an essential activity within health and care settings as well as universities and advances our understanding of how to deliver high-quality patient care. Research activity will not only enhance your job satisfaction but also contribute to the performance of your organisation (NIHR 2024a). It might also help you get a promotion or secure that job you have always wanted. Research is very high on the health and care service agenda of many countries, and significant amounts of public funding are invested in high-quality research.

The concept that practice should be based on research evidence is now universally acknowledged, with practitioners increasingly concerned that the care they deliver is based on the strongest available evidence. This concept, known as evidence-based practice, has become the cornerstone of health care and has been described by Aveyard et al. (2023b: 13) as follows:

> *Put simply, evidence-based practice is practice that is supported by the best available evidence, taking into account the patient's/client's preferences and using your own judgement. If we practise an evidence-based approach, then we are set to give the best possible care.*

From this definition, you can see that evidence-based practice is not just about evidence but also involves professional judgement as well as patient and client preference. If you are interested in the principles that underpin evidence-based practice, then *A Beginner's Guide to Evidence-based Practice in Health and Social Care* (Aveyard et al. 2023b) is a good place to start.

The development of this evidence base is not reliant on large-scale projects alone, although larger projects will tend to have more of an impact. Small-scale research projects are also essential for the following reasons:

- A small-scale project can be the springboard for a larger project as well as serve as a pilot project from which that larger project is developed.
- Small-scale projects provide essential research training, providing the researcher with the knowledge and skills to work on and lead larger-scale projects.
- Undertaking a small project will introduce you to a network of people who can support your subsequent research endeavours.
- Undertaking a small project will enhance your understanding of research more generally.

Small-scale research projects are therefore a great way to initiate or maintain your research interests. A small-scale project is often undertaken as a component of a university course of study, although not necessarily so. You might, for instance, be an independent researcher or be working as part of a group.

In this book, we describe how to undertake a small-scale project. We focus on audits, service evaluations and small-scale research projects – projects that are often undertaken by novice researchers – but much of what we explore is applicable to other types of study. For many of you, your project will have its origins in clinical practice, and your research question will reflect that. As experienced supervisors of students undertaking small-scale projects, including audits and service evaluations, we draw on projects previously undertaken by healthcare education professionals.

We have written this book as a guide to doing a small-scale project, whether that is a small local study, such as an audit or service evaluation, or a project that is part of a postgraduate degree, including doctoral study. We provide an overview of the stages that are involved when undertaking a small-scale project and signpost you to key resources. We discuss the importance of identifying a research question that is both relevant and appropriate to clinical practice and can be answered within the time frame available to you. We will look at suitable research questions and the methods that would be appropriate to address them. We will also look at the practicalities that need to be considered when doing the project.

If you have started to think about your research plans, then you have probably already begun to read around your topic. You probably feel a mixture of anticipation and apprehension about the task ahead. You may be wondering how to make sense of what you are reading and how you might integrate the different types of evidence into your literature review at the level expected of a postgraduate student.

- In Chapter 1 we discuss how you work towards your research question, and ensure that the scope of the project is realistic within the time frame available to you.
- In Chapter 2 we address how you identify and review literature that is relevant for identifying the gap in the knowledge base your research question is directed at.
- In Chapter 3 our focus is on how you plan your project in detail, including how you identify the methods that are appropriate to address your research question.
- In Chapter 4 we turn our attention to the ethical approval and other permissions you will need to secure to proceed with your project, including gatekeeper access to the research site.
- In Chapter 5 we discuss the practicalities of undertaking your project, whether it be an audit, service evaluation or small-scale research project.
- In Chapter 6 we look at different methods of analysis that you might use in a small-scale project.
- Finally, in Chapter 7 we address the writing up and dissemination of your findings.

1

Getting started and identifying the question for your research project

In this book we provide a detailed guide to the stages of undertaking a small-scale research project, by which we mean audit, service evaluation, as well as other types of research project. It will become apparent that in some healthcare systems, audit and service evaluation are not considered 'research' because their findings are specific to the local context and are not generalisable; however, they employ similar methods to those used in research projects. Therefore, when we use the terms 'research' and 'research question', they are generally used to encompass all project types, including audit and service evaluation.

We will focus here on small-scale research projects that you would be likely to undertake for an undergraduate- or master's-level award but this is a guide only; all of the principles outlined in this book are applicable to projects undertaken as part of doctoral study. We anticipate that you will be undertaking your project in the clinical area and that your focus will be to enhance patient care and/or patient or staff experience, or within healthcare education. Hence the project is very likely to have its roots in clinical practice, which we will return to throughout the book.

Audit and service evaluation projects are generally considered to be grounded in the tradition of quality improvement – an initiative to drive quality within health care with a focus on immediate clinical issues and where the findings of a project can be implemented and evaluated in the local setting. Both audit and service evaluation are described as a cycle of activity: a clinical issue is identified and investigated, and the findings are implemented into practice. For example, in the UK, the service evaluation cycle of 'Plan, Do, Study, Act' (Deming 1986) provides a clear guide to the way that clinical problems can be identified and investigated so that local change can happen (see Figure 1.1). Audit follows a similar cycle, except that it also includes reference to a standard or guideline that the observation in practice is compared with (see Figure 1.2).

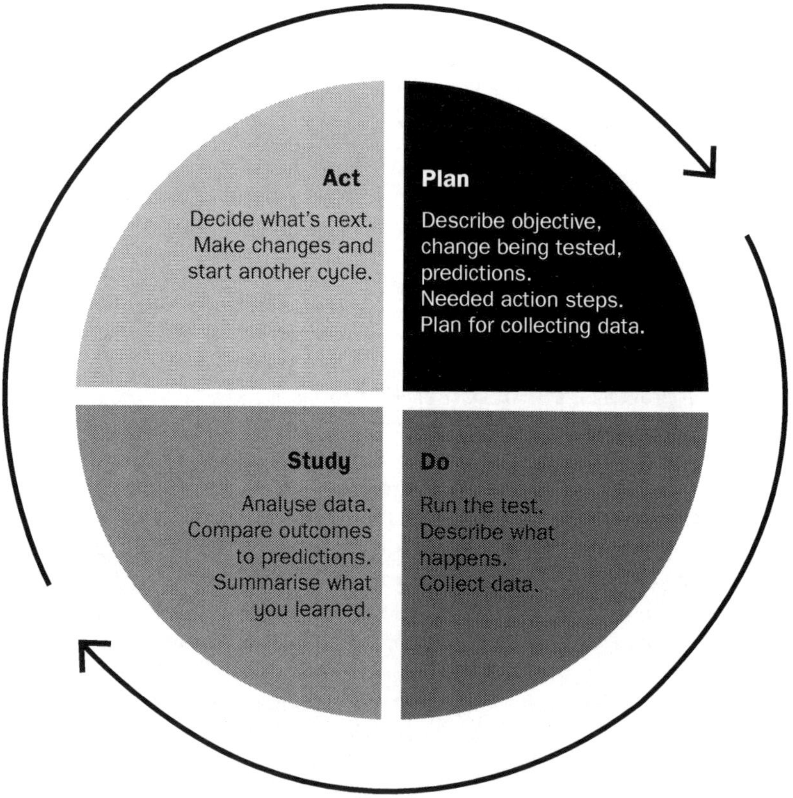

Figure 1.1 The 'Plan, Do, Study, Act' cycle (adapted from Deming 1986)

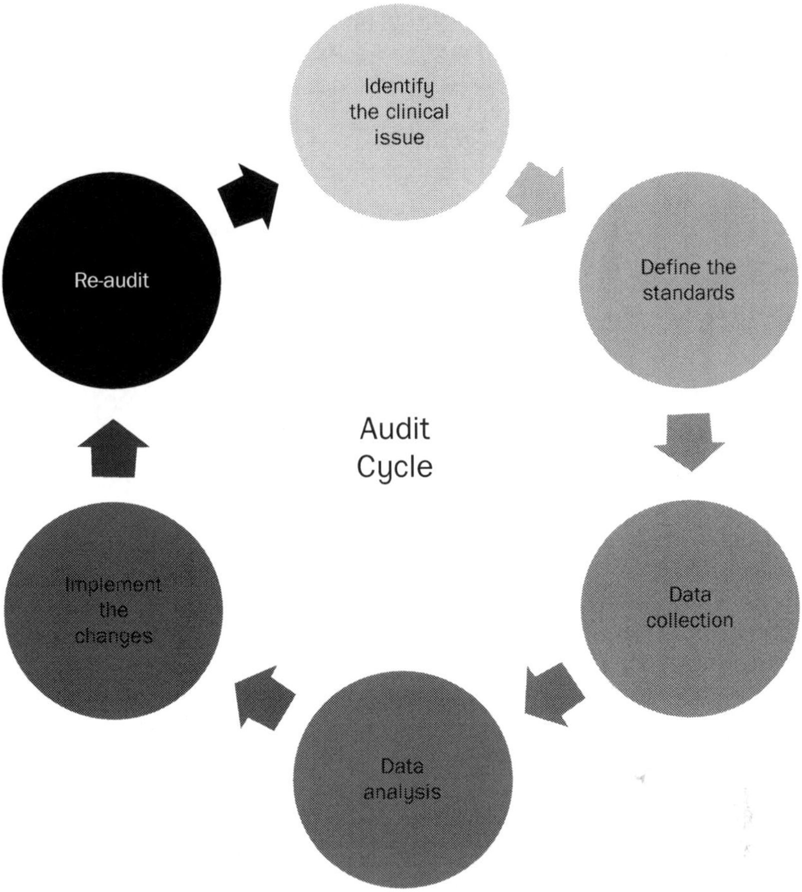

Figure 1.2 Clinical audit cycle (adapted from Limb et al. 2017)

Research, in contrast, is grounded in the tradition of generating new knowledge. As with audit and service evaluation, a problem is identified that requires investigation. However, the problem is not necessarily associated with the clinical setting, although very often it is. As with audit and service evaluation, research projects follow an investigation or method of study but there is not always a corresponding pathway for the implementation of change. These differences need to be borne in mind when you plan your project. In practice, the differences are relatively minor. Whilst the findings from an audit or service evaluation can be fed back into the organisation that initiated them, so too can the findings from research and it is clear all projects aim to improve the service we offer to our patients. Furthermore, all three types – audit, service evaluation and research – draw on the principles of research, including overriding philosophies, traditions and methods.

A summary of research traditions that influence your audit, service evaluation or small-scale research project

For many years and in many disciplines, including health care, the dominant approach or paradigm within which research has been conducted is the 'positivist paradigm'. The term 'positivist paradigm' largely equates to the classic 'scientific paradigm', in which experiments and observations are undertaken in a controlled manner, with precision and accuracy. For example, some geologists study the earth's crust, some geographers measure coastal erosion, and some medical scientists study the development of new antibiotics. The object of their study, be it the earth's crust, coastlines or antibiotics, is definable and measurable. Experiments or observations are undertaken according to a strict protocol that ensures reliability and repeatability. Generally, there is detachment between the scientist and the object or subject being studied. The sample sizes tend to be large and there is an anticipation that the results can be generalised.

We have seen monumental advances in the treatment and management of diseases as a result of research undertaken within the positivist paradigm using quantitative research methods, developments that have revolutionised health care. For example, the drugs used to treat cancer are systematically tested in a series of trials in an attempt to identify effectiveness of the new treatment and further treatments after that. As a new drug is shown to be effective, further trials can be undertaken to determine the dose needed and so on. Studies on new drugs generally start with small-scale studies that determine the toxicity and acceptability of the new drug followed by larger studies where the new drug is carefully compared to the existing drugs available. This is known as a randomised controlled trial (RCT), where the new drug is compared to the standard drug in a carefully controlled experiment where all predetermined outcomes are monitored.

We are fortunate to live in an era when treatments for diseases have been developed and tested in this rigorous way. For example, in the 1970s, scientists did not know whether the best course of action for breast cancer was to remove the lump or the whole breast. Clinical trials (RCTs) were undertaken to compare the two courses of action and it became clear that, for certain tumours, removal of the lump was as effective as removal of the whole breast. Women with breast cancer who agreed to take part were allocated at random to a lumpectomy or full mastectomy and followed up. As a result of randomisation of the women to different groups within trials, any difference in outcome could be attributed to the effect (or lack of effect) of the intervention. The scientists were able to measure survival in terms of months and years to determine whether lumpectomy was as effective as a full mastectomy. Once this was established, fine-tuning of the treatment for breast cancer was made possible by many subsequent RCTs to determine the type and dose of chemotherapy required and so on.

This scientific process has been applied to the vast majority of treatments we use today, many of which are built on years of research evidence. Those patients who agree to participate in trials are, to some extent, stepping into the unknown, since they are asked to forgo standard treatment for a new, alternative form of treatment. Gradually and incrementally over time, each new clinical trial builds on the evidence of previous trials, providing a strong evidence base for the interventions that are used to treat illness and disease.

Despite the rigour associated with RCTs, it was apparent early on that a single RCT was not sufficient in and of itself to make a strong argument to change a treatment. Instead, what was needed was a database of all the available RCTs on a new treatment or intervention. In order to do this, the Cochrane Collaboration was established in 1993, with the aim of amalgamating all relevant studies and providing an overall estimate of the effectiveness of a new treatment or intervention. Combining the results of many studies is more compelling than relying on those of a single study.

The aim of positivist, quantitative research is to generate results that are generalisable to the wider population. The reviews provided by the Cochrane Collaboration and subsequently the Campbell Collaboration and other institutions help shape treatment policy, such as those developed by the National Institute for Health and Care Excellence (NICE), ensuring that there is a clear evidence base for the treatments and care available. Research of this magnitude is generally conducted over a long period of time, by teams of scientists using large sample sizes in order to demonstrate generalisable results: conditions that are far beyond the scope of any master's- or doctoral-level study. However, this does not mean that smaller-scale projects, and those involving methods other than an RCT (such as a survey), cannot be undertaken. An audit of waiting times in a department is one example of a smaller-scale 'pilot' project involving methods of numerical measurement. Using a short questionnaire to survey the service provided in a department is another. These can be undertaken in a systematic way and provide data relevant to a local area and act also as a blueprint for future projects, and most certainly fall into the category of 'good learning'.

You will now be aware that positivist research is well established in our culture and has provided research-based evidence upon which our services are delivered. However, not all research within health and social care can be explored through a positivist approach and not all research that we need within health and social care can be measured numerically. In recent years, there has been an emphasis on the importance of research seen through a different, 'non-numerical' lens. There are many examples of this. Goffman's (1961) observational work of the practices in mental health institutions (then known as asylums) in the 1950s and 1960s is an example of research undertaken through a different lens; a lens that focuses on understanding events and situations as they occur and without numerical measurement. Goffman observed the care delivered on an inpatient mental health unit and documented the institutionalised and routine practices he witnessed that were not focused on individual patient need. Thus Goffman did not employ numerical methods; instead, he observed and interpreted. There are various paradigms for research undertaken through a non-numerical lens, including constructivist or naturalist inquiry. As its name implies, constructivism requires the co-creation of data with the research participant; the researcher helps to shape the data by engagement with the participant in order to fully understand their perspective. Research undertaken within naturalist inquiry reinforces the concept that those undertaking the research do not try to manipulate or change the environment; they observe what is occurring naturally. Research undertaken using this paradigm is often qualitative and associated with achieving an in-depth understanding and exploration of a phenomenon – for example, a patient/client's experience of illness or other complaint. A study undertaken within the constructivist paradigm provides a deep understanding of the experience that the researchers set out to explore in a way that would not be possible by conducting an experiment or by distributing a questionnaire, for example. Goffman's work and that of others has had a clear impact: it has led to changes in social policy and the way people with mental illness are looked after.

In addition to positivism and constructivism, there are other paradigms which shape and influence the way research is undertaken. You might find other paradigms to be a useful lens through which to undertake your project. There are also many research questions that benefit from a combination of different paradigms. Studies which incorporate both quantitative and qualitative research methods are referred to as mixed-methods studies/research. For example, the numerical measurement of the efficacy of a drug might be supplemented by information about why people do or do not find the drug acceptable to take. Thus mixed-methods research draws on the principles from different paradigms. The influence of the underpinning philosophy or paradigm on your subsequent methodology and method for your study is discussed in detail in Chapter 3.

There might be more than one suitable paradigm to guide your project. Projects that fall within the positivist paradigm – normally using quantitative methods – can be undertaken, even if not at the scale that might achieve generalisability. Alternatively, projects that seek understanding and generally require smaller sample sizes – normally using qualitative methods – can also be undertaken. You might also identify a mixed-methods approach as a way forward, based on the advice of your supervisor.

Understanding the core features of audit, service evaluation and small-scale research projects

Despite the different traditions within research, there are some commonalities between projects, regardless of whether your project is an audit, service evaluation or small-scale research project. All research projects (including audit and service evaluation, which we address later) share a similar structure that is well established among the research community and is one that we recommend you follow for your project. This structure first involves the identification of a research question, followed by a method to address that question. The next step consists of the documentation and presentation of your results/findings. Finally, you need to discuss what your results/findings really mean. This structure has long been the format by which research projects are published and disseminated and remains a logical way in which to present your project. It reflects the acronym IMRaD – **I**ntroduction, **M**ethods, **R**esults **a**nd **D**iscussion – and has been the accepted format for academic work over the past sixty years (Sollaci and Pereira 2004; Suhonen 2014). Adhering to this structure will ensure that your project is framed in a way that is familiar to those interested in your work. Following this structure will help you to see how your project differs from the work that others are doing: the differences and similarities should be clear to see and understanding this will help to build your confidence in the project you are doing and how it contributes to the wider picture of research. However, we also recommend that you follow the advice offered by your academic institution regarding the structure and layout of your project.

> If you are unsure about any of this, log into a database with which you are familiar and search for a couple of research papers, preferably from different research traditions. You will identify the following structure to those papers: Aim or Research Question / Introduction / Methods / Results or Findings / Discussion / Conclusion. This is the structure and design you are aiming for when you undertake your audit, service evaluation or small-scale empirical project.

The difference between audit, service evaluation and a small-scale research project

Having emphasised the overall similarities between projects, let us now explore the differences. Whilst an audit is almost certainly aligned with a positivist, quantitative approach, service evaluations and small-scale research projects can be conducted using many different approaches.

Audit

An audit is a project that seeks to identify whether the service provided to patients or clients meets a certain standard. In order to undertake an audit, there needs to be agreed, pre-set standards for the service or care that is provided. These are usually national standards, not those set by a particular unit or hospital. Data is then collected which measures the service or care provision in order to assess whether the national standard set is met and how often. You can see that audit generally follows a positivist/quantitative approach of undertaking numerical measurement to collect data. Sometimes the data collected might be found in the everyday documentation on patient care. At other times, data might be collected using observation, questionnaires or interviews. It is important to note that nothing 'extra' is done in an audit; there are no additional interventions or procedures. Someone undertaking an audit is examining current practice and measuring against an agreed benchmark. If you undertake an audit, you act as the auditor and seek to measure various key indicators that tell us whether the standards that have been set are being met. Audit follows all the same components of a research project as outlined above, even though audit is typically not recognised as 'research' as the results are only relevant to the particular unit in which the audit was undertaken and are therefore not generalisable. Your findings will however be highly relevant to the unit in which you conducted your audit. In addition, as audit is not typically deemed to be research, it is generally not subject to the same governance as research, and the permissions needed to undertake an audit are generally less exacting than for a research project. This makes audit an attractive option for anyone wanting to undertake a small-scale research project as a dissertation or as a standalone project in its own right. For further details, hints and tips about undertaking an audit, we refer you to the Healthcare Quality Improvement Partnership (HQIP) website (hqip.org.uk) and the NHS clinical audit web page (https://www.england.nhs.uk/clinaudit/).

Example 1: You might decide to undertake an audit to determine whether analgesia is given in a timely manner to patients with a fractured neck of femur in the emergency department. National standards for the administration of analgesia exist and these ensure that patients receive timely pain relief as recommended by a committee who have explored optimum practice in detail, hence reducing the workload for individual clinicians. This will include the administration of pain relief on admission to the unit. An audit of the analgesia administered to patients over a given time frame will determine whether all patients received immediate pain relief upon entering the emergency department and hence if the standards are being met.

Example 2: An audit might also be undertaken to determine the extent to which a hospital or university department's research protocols adhere to current Equality, Diversity and Inclusion (EDI) principles. In the UK, the National Institute for Health and Care Research (NIHR 2022) has published standards on equality, diversity and inclusion. These standards ensure that research is not focused on a small proportion of the population but instead aims for equal access to research for all. This helps to ensure that research findings apply to everyone in a community, thereby not perpetuating inequalities. Auditing research protocols for evidence about the application of the principles of Equality, Diversity and Inclusion will help us understand the extent to which the principles are being adopted in our communities.

Service evaluation

Service evaluation is designed to determine the standard of care that is delivered by the service you are providing. You will see the similarity here with audit: both measure (or evaluate) a specific service, and there is no attempt to introduce a new intervention or procedure which can be measured. A service evaluation, as its name suggests, evaluates what is already happening in a service. Either existing data can be collected to measure the service, or questionnaires or interviews can be used to collect additional data. As with audit, patient care will be unaffected.

The difference between an audit and a service evaluation is that for the latter, there is no set standard against which to measure. Hence service evaluations are undertaken to understand the views of patients and clients about the service they receive, without the need for comparison with a specific national standard. Service evaluations are therefore more flexible in their approach than an audit, and can be undertaken to evaluate any type of service, whether or not standards for best practice exist. As such service evaluations can follow either a positivist/quantitative approach or a constructivist/naturalistic/qualitative approach where understanding the perspective of others is key. For further information, see the NHS Evaluation toolkit, available at https://nhsevaluationtoolkit.net/.

Example 1: The local community midwifery team might decide to undertake a service evaluation of the care received by women seeking asylum. There are, at the time of writing, no national standards and care is delivered according to the needs of the woman. However, women seeking asylum are likely to have specific needs and it is important that the professionals providing the service understand what these are and whether the care received is appropriate. The team would be making a local evaluation of the care that is received by women seeking asylum. Their intention would not be to generalise their findings to the wider population but instead to evaluate the experiences of the women in their care and adapt and improve the service accordingly.

Example 2: A service evaluation might also be undertaken to assess the acceptability to patients of extending the provision of nurse-led clinics in primary care; for example, to explore whether clinics established for asthma or diabetes might be applicable to other conditions. Seeking the views of patients attending such clinics would give the researchers an understanding of factors they would need to consider when delivering and extending the scope of nurse-led clinics. It should be noted that patients' views are only one part of the jigsaw and that clinical appropriateness and skill mix should also be considered.

You can see the similarity and differences between audit and service evaluation. Both aim to evaluate a service/delivery of care that is already established, providing results or findings that are relevant to the local community; their findings/results are not generalisable. Therefore, due to the local interest of the project and lack of generalisability they are less likely to be published, although at times understanding the local evaluation of care can be useful to a wider audience and hence the findings worthy of publication.

So, neither audit nor service evaluation fall into the category of 'research'; they aim to evaluate a service rather than to generate 'new knowledge' that is generalisable. Of course, they do generate new knowledge but it will be specific to the service through which the data was generated. The UK Policy Framework for Health and Social Care Research (NHS Health Research Authority 2025) emphasises the difference between audit/service evaluation and research. The authority argues that audit and service improvement projects should not be presented as 'research', nor are they subject to the same standards as research. For the purposes of a small-scale project, the differences are minimal and the need to employ systematic and rigorous processes is applicable across the board. In some countries, the technical difference is significant. For example, in the UK there are different regulatory procedures for audit/service evaluation and research. Research is subject to full ethical scrutiny whereas audit/service evaluation are often subject to a less vigorous review (we will discuss this in more detail in Chapter 4). In some other countries, however, only studies that propose to evaluate a new intervention are subject to close ethical scrutiny (Grazioli et al. 2024). Researchers need therefore to be mindful of the local context so that they obtain the correct ethical approval and other permissions.

In this book, we take the position that given audit, service evaluation and research essentially utilise the same methods – and hence the learning inherent to audit/service evaluation is similar to that of research – there is an advantage to undertaking projects that are subject to less formal governance, if these can be achieved within a shorter time frame. Of course, the conduct of a service evaluation or audit should adhere to the highest of ethical standards; however, as Grazioli et al. (2024) explain, these are governed with reference to professional standards rather than explicit and formal ethical scrutiny.

Small-scale research projects

Small-scale research projects are an alternative to an audit or service evaluation. Such a project might be described as an 'empirical project' or a 'clinical research project': these terms are often used interchangeably, with a clinical research project undertaken in the clinical area. Clinical research is defined differently by different organisations. For example, the National Institute for Health and Care Research refers to clinical research as 'patient orientated research' (NIHR 2024b) in which the investigator interacts with those participating in the project. In contrast, the US National Institute on Aging (2023) defines clinical research as the 'study of health and illness in people' and whose remit is not restricted to patients. Likewise, the NHS Health Research Authority (2024) states that clinical research 'aims to find out about an illness, condition, treatment, therapy or care by directly involving people'. Johns Hopkins University (2025) defines clinical research as 'the comprehensive study of the safety and effectiveness of the most promising advances in patient care'. We can see some clear differences in definitions of the term clinical research. Some are fairly broad and involve the study of health and illness in people, whereas others are more specific. Therefore, it is difficult to be precise about the meaning of the term 'clinical research'. We argue that 'research' is a more useful umbrella term that embraces research done both in the clinical area as well as in other settings such as education. In this book, we focus on small-scale empirical studies that might have application in clinical practice or in an educational setting; in view of this, we use the term small-scale research project to refer to all types of research project referred to here.

A small-scale research project differs from an audit or service evaluation in its aim: to generate new knowledge rather than to evaluate an existing system. The difference, however, is subtle and it could be argued that both audit and service evaluation advance knowledge about the system they seek to evaluate. The important point here is that research aims to produce knowledge that is generalisable. However, the results or findings of a small-scale research project are likely to be preliminary in nature and hence their generalisability will be limited. To complicate things further, there is some debate within qualitative research as to the generalisability of the results: qualitative researchers often use the term 'transferable' rather than 'generalisable'. This debate has been informed by Lincoln and Guba (1985), who argue that generalisability does not apply to qualitative research due to the small sample size involved and the localised nature of the development of knowledge. Instead, they propose the concept of transferability, meaning that the findings of a qualitative research study are transferable to other areas. This could be considered to be a form of generalisability not applicable to audit or service evaluation. The difference is so subtle that many might query whether the results of any small-scale research project, audit or service evaluation are truly generalisable.

The key point is that anyone undertaking small-scale research (rather than an audit or service evaluation) is seeking to generate knowledge – even if this is achieved in a very modest way –and is generalisable or at least transferable. The findings or results from the study are predicted to be applicable beyond the immediate clinical area in which they were obtained and publication of the results might be realistic. It is important to note that for a small-scale research project, it is likely to be regarded as a pilot or feasibility study, although both of these are publishable in their own right. There are many resources to help you understand small-scale research projects and we will refer to these throughout, but a good start might be Thomas (2023).

Example 1: One example of a small-scale research project is a study that was undertaken in northern India (Stewart 2020). The student researcher obtained funding to explore how and when patients in a local hospital in northern India sought treatment from the local healthcare provider and when they relied on traditional medicine instead. Aware of the many financial and cultural influences on health-seeking behaviour, the student researcher was interested in understanding when and why hospital care was accessed by those who participated in the study.

You can see that this project is not specific to any particular healthcare unit or environment; the student researcher did not seek to evaluate a service. Instead, they were seeking to understand health-seeking behaviour in a culture very different to their own. Clearly an ambitious study for a small-scale project but undertaken in a robust manner, it provides some preliminary data on this topic. For this reason, the study fits into the category of small-scale research.

Example 2: Another example of a small-scale research project is a study that was undertaken to explore the way in which nurses provide information to patients prior to nursing care procedures (Aveyard et al. 2022). This study was developed from earlier work. Aveyard et al. recruited a small sample of qualified nurses to the study in order to describe incidents in which consent had or had not been obtained prior to nursing care procedures in order to understand how informed consent is currently sought.

In the example above, the researchers were not evaluating a service, but instead exploring how nursing care is delivered. They were seeking an understanding of the way nursing care is delivered and which might be generalisable or transferable. This study did result in a publication (Aveyard et al. 2022). It is also useful to note that a study involving nurses does not necessarily need to be undertaken within a clinical context – Aveyard et al. conducted their study in a university environment. Although the study focused on a clinical area, the participants were students undertaking a post-registration module or course. It was classified as research and all the necessary permissions were obtained to undertake the study.

It could be argued that a similar study to that of Aveyard et al. (2022) could have been conducted as a service evaluation. The expectation that nurses should obtain informed consent is an established standard within health care and a requirement of all local Trusts. Hence it would be appropriate to evaluate the service in order to identify the extent to which information is given prior to obtaining informed consent in a particular clinical area. This illustrates the sometimes-blurred boundary between research and service evaluation. The difference is often subtle, and in some countries there may be no distinction whatsoever. If you are intending to publish your service evaluation, you will need to demonstrate compliance with relevant governance procedures.

Using secondary sources

There are alternative ways to tackle a small-scale project. Undertaking a literature review often comes to mind when using secondary sources. This is discussed in a separate publication (Aveyard et al. 2026) and will not be referred to in detail here. However, there are many other types of secondary sources that could be reviewed for a small-scale research project. For example, you might decide to review a series of television programmes to examine how the treatment of individuals with a specific condition is portrayed on television and how realistically the illness is documented (thanks to Stephie Asbridge for this). To do this, you could settle down to watch the requisite programmes, although that might be rather time-consuming!

Secondary sources can be used in many ways. Datasets might be available to you from existing projects or from sources from which you can obtain information. Examples of the use of secondary data are provided by Dodds et al. (2021). Another source of secondary data is to use Freedom of Information (FoI) requests for research purposes (Yale et al. 2024). For example, a student was interested in comparing the guidelines produced by different maternity services for the use of water births for women who had had a previous caesarean section. Guidelines were obtained from each of the different maternity services nationally and were compared in order to establish national differences and similarities in practice from the guidelines available.

Research or project – which is the correct term?

We have briefly outlined the possible different methods for doing your small-scale project. It is important that you understand the differences and then identify the type of project you wish to undertake. In addition, terms are often used interchangeably. If you are doing an audit or service evaluation project, you might choose to omit the term 'research' and simply state 'project' or 'project question'. This ensures that you demonstrate your awareness of the differences between the possible projects and the specific remits of research, audit and service evaluation. However, you are unlikely to be challenged if you refer to your project as 'research' as long as you have followed the correct procedures and obtained the correct permissions. In this book, the terms 'project' and 'research' are used to refer to audit, service evaluation, as well as other types of research project. In the UK, the Health Research Authority has a decision tree which you can use to check which approach your project fits and which permissions are needed (this is discussed further in Chapter 4). It is up to you and your supervisor to agree between you the approach you will adopt. Once you have agreed upon this, return to the structure that is followed by almost all small-scale research projects, audits and service evaluations: Aim or Research Question / Introduction / Methods / Results or Findings / Discussion / Conclusion.

Identifying your question

All projects require a clearly focused question. There is a lot written about question development prior to a research study and it is important to note that it is not an exact science, but there are instead a number of guiding principles. Common consensus suggests that questions need to be focused, not over-ambitious, sufficiently interesting to retain your interest, and doable within the time frame available to you.

There are tools to help identify your question, including PICO (Population, Intervention, Comparison, Outcome), whose origins can be traced to the early discussion about evidence-based practice (Richardson and Murphy 1998) and the idea that good research questions generally contain three or four well-defined elements. The traditional PICO tool (Fineout-Overholt and Johnston 2005) has also been adapted for qualitative research questions: PICO (**P**opulation, **I**ssue, **C**ontext, **O**utcome). There are other tools, many of which have a dual aim – to develop the question and to develop the subsequent search strategy – so be aware of this when trying to identify a tool to use.

Use of a tool will not identify a question but can help to shape one. A tool will help to ensure the question is suitably focused but you need to have an idea of your topic and developing question. It is our view that many good questions come from clinical or educational practice – either something identified from your practice or something that is recommended to you by a colleague. This ensures that the question is grounded in the realities of clinical or educational practice rather than an abstract idea. It also ensures that once the project is finished you can feed your findings back into the practice area for the direct benefit of patients/clients or the workforce. The process for doing so is implicit when doing an audit or service evaluation as this is an expectation of the project. Furthermore, the focus of the project will have been identified or experienced by colleagues in the practice area.

In this book, we refer to examples of student projects – audits, service evaluations and research projects – to illustrate the various stages of the research process. Below we provide some examples of projects where we list the topic followed by the focused question, together with alternatives that would have altered the focus of the project. We have identified a question for each of audit, service evaluation and research project. All of these questions arose from concerns from a practice context.

First, a student who was working in the ear, nose and throat (ENT) department became aware of the complications that sometimes arise if otitis externa is not managed appropriately and hence the importance that it is managed according to the evidence as summarised in the guidelines. The student identified the following question for an audit:

Topic: How do we manage otitis externa in ENT?
Research question (for an audit): Is the current management of patients with Otitis Externa in the local ENT department meeting the standards set out in the NICE (2024) guidelines and the local ear swabbing protocol? (adapted from Ferreira 2025)

Another student became interested in the services offered to older adults in a community day centre and wanted to evaluate the benefits of these in a service evaluation:

Topic: The evaluation of a community day centre
Research question (for a service evaluation): Do the services offered for older adult users at a community day centre meet their needs? (adapted from Birch 2024)

The following student undertook an enquiry into the provision of social services for asylum seekers but did this as a small-scale research project rather than a service evaluation. This project was exploratory rather than evaluative and hence was undertaken as a small-scale research project:

Topic: Examination of social services support for asylum-seeking families in England (adapted from Pugh 2023)
Research question: How do social workers in a local area support asylum-seeking women with pre-school-age children?

You will have observed that in some of the questions, the population is well defined – for example, 'asylum-seeking women' – and in others it is less well defined – for example, 'older adult users'. There is no right or wrong here; it depends on the needs of your project and how focused your question needs to be. You will also see that there is a context and in some cases a measurable outcome. Again, there is no right or wrong here; the scope of the question is a matter of judgement.

Getting the question right is your first priority. Being over-ambitious is one of the most common errors a student can make when embarking on a project. The research process is detailed and you will not be able to give it the attention required if your project is too large. A question that is over-ambitious will not be answerable in the time frame available and you are likely to end up writing an essay about the topic and not achieving your goal. Furthermore, you are likely to be working as a lone researcher with no colleagues to outsource tasks to: you will have a supervisory team but their role will be advisory, not 'hands on'. Therefore, this will limit the size and scope of the project. Setting a question that is not ambitious enough is a less common error but important to bear in mind. Such a question might lead you to an insufficient number of participants, resulting in a very limited dataset. Your supervisor will guide you on the appropriate focus for your research question but do bear in mind that the tendency is often to be ambitious rather than realistic about what can be achieved in the time frame, with the depth and rigour that is required.

Identifying your question will likely be an iterative process and the research question will determine the way in which the study will be undertaken and vice versa. You might have an idea for a project and undertake an initial review of the literature (as we discuss in Chapter 2), and identify that there is already a large body of knowledge on the subject but there is a subset of literature that might indicate a topic that would be worthy of further exploration. You would then decide to refocus your question. Your question might also be shaped by practical considerations about how you will collect data. You need to keep what is practical firmly in mind when undertaking a small-scale project as you will not have the resources to pursue anything too ambitious.

Box 1.1: Using the term 'research question'

Note that the term 'research question' is often used when undertaking audit and service evaluation even though it might not be classified as 'research'. This is because all projects follow a logical systematic process and the differences between the projects are very small indeed.

Identifying a 'gap in knowledge'

In addition to their origins in clinical and professional practice, good research questions also need to identify a 'gap in knowledge'. This simply means that there is inadequate or missing information about a clinical or educational context that your project might address. For those undertaking an audit or service evaluation, the 'gap in knowledge' or understanding is likely to be identified by professionals working in clinical practice who need to know that a service is working to an agreed or acceptable standard. For those of you doing a small-scale research project, the 'gap in knowledge' can be determined when you cannot find an answer to a question in the existing literature – by doing a literature search.

Prior to any research study, audit or service evaluation, you need to establish what is currently known about the topic you are interested in. It is important to know what research has been undertaken in the area, and to determine if a similar study has already been done. If that is the case, the strength of evidence will depend on the size and quality of the earlier study, when it was conducted and whether its results are generalisable – that is, applicable to populations outside the study itself. Therefore, identifying a similar study does not necessarily mean that you should not repeat it. What is important is that you can recognise this and understand how your own study might contribute. It is therefore important to understand the research that has already been undertaken in an area in order to assess any gap in knowledge. For an audit or service evaluation, you will need to understand why the practice you are auditing is important. A short literature review will usually be included in the introduction to a study, summarising the existing knowledge in the area and justifying the study that is about to be reported. We will discuss this in detail in Chapter 2.

Defining the terms you use in the question for your project

A vital part of setting your research question is to ensure that all the terms you refer to are clearly defined so that both you and your readers are clear about the focus of your study and that there is no possibility of 'drift' in terms of its scope.

Often, the terms used within a question are easily defined. Take, for example, 'handwashing'. This term probably means the same thing to most people and a simple definition will suffice. Other terms will require a more detailed definition. As another example, take the concept of 'spirituality'. Understanding a patient or client's need for spiritual connection is a common aspiration within health and social care. However, spirituality is not easy to define, meaning that this concept is very difficult to research. A researcher has two options here: either identify and adopt a definition of spirituality that they are happy to refer to consistently in their project, *or* take a concept that is often associated with spirituality that is more easily definable and alter the focus of the project. The point here is that all of the terms you use need to be clearly defined; otherwise, you risk losing the thread and the remit of your project.

Other terms are neither straightforward nor complex but nonetheless require definition. For example, imagine you are exploring how constant observations are managed in a mental health setting. Constant observations might seem like a clearly defined concept but there are different forms of observation: constant observation and intermittent observation to name but two, and indeed these might not be used consistently. The researcher therefore needs to be very clear about the type of observation they are referring to in their project – and not be tempted to include other types of observation in the study once the focus is decided on.

For some researchers, undertaking a concept analysis can be a useful step in ensuring clarity in the terms they use. This can undoubtedly be a useful exercise but is likely to be beyond the scope of someone doing a small-scale project. Other options for concept clarification are available and we have discussed these in detail in a separate publication (Mounce et al. 2025).

Choosing your method

All projects have a clearly defined method. This will include reference to the approach chosen (i.e. audit, service evaluation or small-scale research project), followed by a detailed exploration of the steps needed to undertake the project. When you look at examples of small-scale projects, these will include a clear description of where the research was undertaken (whilst not identifying the specific clinical area in any way), who was involved and what research methods were used. These might be interviews, focus groups, observation, questionnaires or documentary analysis. The rationale for the use of any of these methods should also be outlined. We discuss the methods you might use in more detail in later chapters of this book. In a separate publication (Aveyard et al. 2025), we present a critical appraisal of ten published studies which illustrate some of the methods you might use in your project. It is important to note that the methods used to address your question are not specific to any particular type of project; that is, audits, service evaluations and small-scale research projects employ a similar array of research methods.

Box 1.2: Artificial intelligence

You may be interested in whether – and how – the wide range of artificial intelligence (AI) tools and software now available might help you undertake project tasks efficiently. There are tools that will search for, retrieve, appraise and summarise information, including academic papers, with varying degrees of accuracy and depth. Whilst these might have some merit in developing your understanding of an area, or even an individual paper, do remember that the quality of what AI retrieves is variable and sometimes completely erroneous.

There are various ways you can use AI to help your learning; for example, you can check your own appraisal of a paper against that provided by an AI tool. We would caution against using AI to 'do' the critical appraisal as the purpose of appraisal is to understand the study rather than to achieve an appraisal. Furthermore, use of AI is not an alternative to the intellectual work that is required in academic study and through which real learning takes place. For these reasons, we recommend that if you use AI, you use it with caution.

Also, be aware that AI software may not be General Data Protection Regulation (GDPR) compliant, meaning data you upload using such software may be stored, used or further distributed. This is particularly important in relation to use of your project data, and what you will have promised your participants with regards to data protection.

Finally, if you do choose to use AI (appropriately), you should make it clear in your write-up where and how AI was used.

We hope this overview of the steps undertaken in all three types of project reinforce the message that there are more similarities than differences between them, whatever different methods and approaches might be used. That is, all researchers are anchored into a recognised process and adhering to this process helps to keep you on track with your project.

In summary

In this chapter, we have explored the similarities and differences between audits, service evaluations and small-scale research projects and how you might identify which is most relevant for you. As you get started, you need to identify a suitable question and possible method by which you will answer the question. Neither the question nor the method is set in stone at this stage; they are often dependent on confirmation by stakeholders who have invested in your project. They are also dependent on what the existing research and wider literature tells you about what we already know about the question you have set yourself, which we discuss in Chapter 2.

Key points

- Small-scale research projects, audits and service evaluations are a great way to introduce yourself to research methods.
- All studies provide a useful way to learn about research, whether or not the method is categorised as 'research'.
- All small-scale projects require a very focused question that needs careful development.
- Small-scale research projects, audits and service evaluations all use the same structure: question, methods, results/findings, discussion.
- The findings of your project are likely to be tentative but will benefit your clinical area or workplace.

2

Doing the literature review

Before you start your audit, service evaluation or other small-scale research project, some detailed engagement with the existing literature is required. This generally falls into two categories:

- Introduction and background
- Literature review

First, you need to explore the background rationale for your question. This information usually forms the basis for your introductory/background chapter, where you discuss the information needed to understand the context for your study. There might be key events that contribute to your understanding of your study or a timeline that helps the reader understand the background and context of your research question. In considering the scope of your project, you will also need to include definitions of the terms you are using.

The next step is the literature review. The aim of the literature review is to focus on the key papers that are *most closely* related to your research question and which illustrate the gap in knowledge you have identified (for small-scale research projects), or that justify why the project is important or why the practice is difficult to implement (for audit and service evaluation). Identifying the studies that are closely related to your overall research question enables you to understand exactly what research has been undertaken in relation to the topic you are interested in – the research that relates most closely to the research/project question you have chosen. Analysis and synthesis of these research papers will enable you to understand what is known in relation to your project and hence what the gap in knowledge is that your project or research will address.

It is the literature review that we will focus on in this chapter. Elsewhere, we make a distinction between 'standalone' literature reviews and those that are undertaken as a prerequisite to an empirical study (Aveyard et al. 2026). A standalone literature review provides a summary of the existing literature that has been published on a particular topic: the emphasis being on what we already know. It can be a substantial piece of work and might constitute a publication in its own right. A literature review that is undertaken prior to a small-scale research project, audit or service evaluation, on the other hand, has a slightly different aim: to identify the gap in knowledge upon which you have based your project (small-scale research project) or why a practice is undertaken and what the barriers might be (audit or service evaluation). In practice, although the method used to undertake a literature review is generally the same, be aware of the subtle differences between the different types of review. When the review is a prerequisite to a larger study, your review might be suitable for publication. For anyone embarking on a master's or undergraduate degree, the time frame and therefore depth of the review often means that this is less likely to be the case, although not improbable. In all circumstances, however, the review remains an essential component to provide evidence as to why your study is important. Literature reviews of all types follow the same generic principles, which we will outline below.

For those of you undertaking a small-scale research project, you should consider your overall research question as provisional until you have undertaken your literature review – you will use the existing literature to refine and reframe your question. This is because what you identify in the literature will almost certainly reshape your question. Your question will evolve as you identify the research that is most connected to your initial research idea. For example, although you may have a question in mind, after some initial searching you may uncover research that you had not anticipated existed. This illustrates how forming a research question is rarely straightforward and that the literature provides more than just a background – a literature review shapes the development of your research question.

If you are undertaking an audit or service evaluation, your research question is most likely to have been identified by someone else – for example, a clinician or manager in your clinical specialty, although you might well have been involved in the process. In this case, the 'gap in knowledge' will be a gap in our understanding as to whether the service in question is adhering to the standards set. In your literature review, you can therefore explore the rationale or evidence base for these standards of practice. Do they emanate from research? Are there evidence-based guidelines that endorse the standards? Is the evidence base well established? What are the barriers to implementation? The answers to these questions will affect the way your project develops. In order to undertake an audit, you need to identify existing national guidelines that justify the current standards. However, these guidelines will be underpinned by evidence and it is important to highlight this.

Let us now look at an example of how you might approach a literature review for a small-scale research project, audit or service evaluation, based on constant observations in a mental health setting. The review could have a different focus, depending on the type of project you undertake:

- For a *small-scale research project*: 'How do clinicians make decisions about the process of setting up constant observations for a patient or client in their care?'
- For a *service evaluation*: 'How do patients or clients experience the process of constant observations?'
- For an *audit*: 'Does the practice of constant observations meet the national guidelines?'

The introduction/background will be very similar for all three types of project. You will explore what is meant by constant observations, explain why they are used, why they are different from intermittent observations, who uses them, and so on. You need to ensure that the definitions you adopt are clear and if there are any competing definitions; if a term might have more than one meaning, you need to acknowledge this.

The literature review for each, however, would be different. For a small-scale research project, you would focus on what is already known from existing research about the management of constant observations: this might include decision-making, insight from colleagues who administer the observations, and so on. The research papers on the management of constant observations you identify will form the basis of your literature review.

> *Literature review question for a small-scale research project:* 'How are constant observations managed in mental health practice?'

For those of you undertaking a service evaluation or audit, you might focus your review on the evidence that underpins the use of constant observations. It is important to note, however, that outcomes of audits and service evaluations are not often published. As discussed earlier, this is because these are smaller-scale projects whose results and findings are applicable to the local setting in which they were undertaken. Therefore, you are more likely to rely on larger-scale published research projects that justify the practice standards rather than local evaluations. Larger research projects that focus on the question posed by your audit or service evaluation will provide data that speaks to the wider generalisable context of the care delivery you are interested in. They will set the context for your research and illustrate national or international concerns: if there are national or international concerns about a specific area, then there are likely to be local concerns too, which is why you identified the topic for audit or service evaluation in the first place.

> *Literature review question for an audit or service evaluation:* 'What is the evidence base or rationale for undertaking constant observations?' Or: 'Why might constant observations be difficult to implement?'

It is of utmost importance that you have a clear focus for your literature review. Although the question for your literature review might be different to the question for your overall project – although it might be similar – its clarity will enable you to write a focused review that is relevant and applicable to your project.

Stages of a literature review

The methods for undertaking a literature review have developed significantly in recent years and so the way we do a literature review prior to a small-scale research project, audit or service evaluation has evolved also. Previously, a literature review might have been little more than a collection of papers that you discussed at the start of your project. This was often an unstructured process that allowed papers, which might have supported the pre-held views of the researcher, to be 'cherry picked' and may not have been representative of the actual body of research.

More recently, the approach to doing a literature review has become more systematic. Even if your literature review is a prerequisite to a larger project, you will be expected to undertake the review in a logical and systematic way and to document this in your project. Do check what is required by your organisation, as some will expect more depth in the review than others and you should plan your review accordingly. As a general rule, your literature review ought to take up to 10–20 per cent of your overall project, so do plan accordingly and proportionately depending on your word count.

The development of methods for doing a literature review has arisen in part as a result of the influence of the Cochrane Collaboration systematic review (Higgins et al. 2024): a systematic, comprehensive and transparent way of undertaking a review, where the aim is to summarise the evidence for the effectiveness of an intervention or drug. This method enables the systematic evaluation of evidence in a way that is logical and detailed, ensuring that priority is given to better-quality evidence, whilst avoiding the temptation to 'cherry pick' papers for discussion in a review. Researchers are required to identify whether the papers in a review provide robust evidence about the effectiveness of an intervention or drug. Cochrane Collaboration reviews quickly became the 'gold standard': known for being thorough and reliable, patients and healthcare staff were given the evidence about which drugs or treatments 'worked' and which did not. It has been said that the Cochrane Collaboration is one of the greatest developments in health care in recent decades.

Cochrane's systematic and comprehensive way of conducting a review is reflected in the development of other methods for undertaking such a task – in particular for qualitative and mixed-methods research and for quantitative reviews where a meta-analysis is not possible. There are now many published methods that outline how to undertake different types of review (e.g. an integrative review), enabling researchers to display rigour and reliability in the process. As a consequence, this has also resulted in a proliferation of methods for doing a review, as documented by Aveyard and Bradbury-Jones (2019) – together with a certain amount of confusion. For example, an overview of methods identified more than 35 different terms for doing a literature review (Aveyard and Bradbury-Jones 2019) and other publications have reported even more. If your review is a prerequisite to a larger study, whether or not you adhere to one of these methods will depend in part on your word count and the requirements of your course of study. As a guide, a scoping review or meta-aggregation might be an appropriate way for you to proceed.

As discussed earlier, the detail in which you undertake a review depends on the size of your overall project. If your review is a minor component of a small-scale project, it will be less detailed than if it were a 'standalone' review or a prerequisite to a larger study. However, no matter the scope of your review, you should use a systematic and logical approach. There are features common to all literature reviews – principles that also apply to doing a 'lighter touch' literature review prior to an audit, service evaluation or small-scale research project. Whatever your project, you will be expected to be rigorous and thorough within the time frame you have. Here, we outline the principles for doing this which you can adapt and apply to your own project as appropriate.

There are four main components of a literature review that will help you to be rigorous: formulating a review question, identifying relevant papers, determining the quality of those papers, and their analysis and synthesis. We will address each of these in the remainder of the chapter.

Formulating a review question

A clear review question is the first requirement of all projects. We use the term 'review question' to distinguish it from a 'research question'. For anyone undertaking a small-scale research project, the review question usually leads to a review of the empirical research that has been undertaken within that particular specialty. Undertaking an initial search of the literature will enable you to identify existing research and whether your research question has already been answered or partially addressed. This initial search will indicate whether you need to adapt your existing, though provisional, question for your project. In addition to perfecting your research question, this approach will help to ensure that your literature review has a specific focus and is distinct from your introduction and background. Furthermore, you need to be clear about the scope and purpose of your review, otherwise you will not be able to identify which research is relevant to your review.

Box 2.1: Research question or review question?

There is potential for confusion here, as there are likely to be two questions to any project you undertake. The first is the overriding research question, as we discussed in Chapter 1. This is the main focus of your project. The second is the question you pose for your literature review. You need to set yourself a review question to guide your literature review, otherwise it risks a lack of focus. In practice, these questions are very likely to be identical, or nearly identical – you search the literature for research papers that address your review question, which then identifies a gap in knowledge that your project seeks to address. However, there are occasions when the question you set for your literature review is slightly different and leads you to a subset of literature. And in a large-scale project, there might be more than one literature review. Furthermore, the term 'comprehensive' with regard to your review is potentially misleading: you do not require comprehensive coverage of all things related to your project. The 'comprehensive' nature of the review means being focused on the review question rather than the review being a comprehensive overview of the topic in general.

For those of you undertaking an audit or service evaluation, a clear question for the review is also needed but the aim of your review will be to explore the evidence base for the care that is being evaluated or to identify barriers to the provision of care. You will be seeking to identify the body of knowledge that justifies the 'prescribed' care delivery. In the event that no such evidence base is identified, this will inform your discussion section.

In the interests of clarity, the use of inclusion and exclusion criteria will help guide the focus of your review. Inclusion and exclusion criteria should be developed with close reference to the review question. Some inclusion criteria will be pragmatic, such as the language of publication (English language only) or year of publication – for example, if you are only interested in papers published after a certain date, such as following the introduction of a new intervention or policy.

The most important inclusion criteria, however, are those that define exactly what you are looking for. The clearer you can be about this, the better. For example, for the small-scale research project regarding the use of constant observations in acute mental health settings above, the main inclusion criterion would be: research papers that explore how constant observations are managed in mental health settings. And for an audit or service evaluation, the main inclusion criterion would be: research papers that provide evidence for the effectiveness of constant observations. This is important as it focuses your thoughts on what you need to find to answer your review question. Then, when you search the available databases and come across an interesting but irrelevant paper, you can be confident of discarding it. If you are in any doubt, consult the methods section of other review papers to see how they handled inclusion and exclusion criteria.

Using a tool to develop the review question

In Chapter 1, we identified tools that can be used to develop a research question. These can also be used to develop a specific question for your review. Examples of different tools are provided by Aveyard et al. (2026) and Cooke et al. (2012).

These tools are not essential for developing a research question for a literature review ahead of a service evaluation, audit or small-scale research study, but they do provide a useful guide. It is important to remember that – as with the overriding question for your project – none of the tools will help you to identify a question if you do not already have something in mind; however, they will assist you in having a very clear focus or remit for a question once one has been identified. If you do not use a specific tool, it is important you identify a literature review question that is relevant and appropriate to your project and that is focused enough so that you do not become inundated with research papers that are not useful to your project.

Searching for literature

Once you have settled on your question, the next step is to search for evidence that enables you to answer it. For anyone undertaking a small-scale research project, the key point is for your search to be 'comprehensive'. This means that you seek to identify all the key literature (usually research) that closely aligns with your literature review question and meets your inclusion criteria. When you search comprehensively, your aim is to identify all the literature rather than a subset of it. This will result in a review that is balanced, rather than based on a 'biased' selection of literature. It prevents the 'cherry picking' of papers. You therefore need to search **and retrieve papers from** the whole body of literature rather than identify a small number of studies **cherry picked** from a larger pool of studies. We understand that this is a big ask for a small-scale research project and that it would be easier to conduct a limited search to make the task more manageable. For anyone undertaking an audit or service evaluation, you do not need to identify the whole body of evidence that justifies a treatment or care pathway – you can be selective but you must highlight the way in which you identified papers. If you are looking for evidence of effectiveness of a standard, you might limit your search to randomised controlled trials which provide evidence on that standard. If you are looking for evidence of patient satisfaction, you might limit your search to qualitative studies, and so on. Do try to think of the boundaries to your search, recorded in your inclusion criteria, so that the literature review feels structured and logical.

The main task when searching for literature is to identify your key search terms. For each key term, you need to identify all the words that mean the same thing, otherwise known as 'synonyms'. An appropriate use of artificial intelligence is the identification of alternative key terms – but do check that you agree with the suggestions generated!

Identifying synonyms ensures that you identify all papers that are relevant to you but which are indexed under a different term. Do bear in mind that terms go in and out of fashion and might be used differently in different countries. You will miss papers if you do not use all appropriate synonyms. However, some synonyms might be too broad and will facilitate the retrieval of inappropriate papers, so you will need to make a judgement here.

Synonyms are combined with the Boolean operator OR. For example,

> mental health OR psychiatry OR mental illness OR …

This ensures that all these terms are identified in papers when you search a database. Your first string of key term + synonyms is likely to be fairly long and will result in hundreds (if not thousands!) of hits. However, when you search your next key term string + synonyms plus AND, the number of hits will reduce enormously as one term from both sets of key terms + synonyms is required for a paper to be identified. For this reason, it is recommended that you use the minimum number of key terms. For example, key terms indicated below:

> How are **constant observations** (+ synonyms) managed in a **mental health** (+ synonyms) setting?

> constant observations **OR** special observations **AND** mental health **OR** psychiatric

You will find much detailed advice on how to search the literature both in textbooks (Aveyard 2023; Aveyard et al. 2026) and online, however you are also advised to access a healthcare librarian if such a service is offered at your institution.

Understanding what you are looking for

If you have formulated a question for your review, the key skill is to identify the literature that addresses it. Your inclusion criteria are the main guide here. If your introduction/background forms its own section in your review – which we recommend – it is vital that the review includes *only* the papers that are most relevant to it. For the vast majority of reviews, research studies will be most important. As discussed in Chapter 1, research is identifiable by the way in which it is presented: you would expect to see a research question or aim followed by a method, results/findings, discussion and conclusion. A piece of research is usually written up as a scientific paper and published in an academic journal and is accessible via a subject-specific database, which we will outline later in this chapter. The types of research paper you need – for example, surveys, questionnaires, qualitative studies – depends on your inclusion criteria, as discussed previously. Your inclusion criteria dictate what is important to your literature review. We do not recommend including any literature reviews within your review; **these are likely to mean that some studies are double counted or inadvertently included twice**. We recommend you focus on primary research only:

- For small-scale research studies, identify research that has looked at the same or a very similar question; the aim is to find out what we already know about your question.
- For audit or service evaluation, identify research that provides evidence for the service you are investigating; the aim is to find out what the existing evidence base is to justify and/or what the barriers are to providing this service.

You may have heard of the term 'hierarchy of evidence', a system in which research methods are ranked according to a hierarchy or order, depending on the likelihood of bias in a study. The implication is that the higher up the hierarchy a methodology is, the stronger the evidence. This is why randomised controlled trials are higher up the hierarchy than qualitative studies, because the former are highly controlled and the latter much less so. However, for questions that seek understanding, qualitative studies are of far more use than randomised controlled trials. Therefore, the term 'hierarchy of evidence' requires an understanding of the research question and what research is needed to understand a particular research question. Therefore, as discussed elsewhere (Aveyard 2023), it is best not to equate the term 'hierarchy of evidence' with a 'hierarchy of studies to include in your review'. The term 'hierarchy of evidence' can be misleading, as it is tempting to think that those methods at the top of the hierarchy will *always* be preferable to those further down it. And this is not the case.

> **Box 2.2: Which evidence is best for your review?**
> If you are looking to explore patients' experience of a new service delivery, you might prioritise your search for qualitative interview studies above questionnaires in the expectation that the former might provide a better understanding of the experience.

Identifying relevant databases

There are a large number of specific healthcare databases. It is important to check which are most relevant to you. Commonly used databases include Medline, CINAHL and PsychInfo but others might also be relevant. We recommend that you start searching one database – ideally the one with which you are most familiar – and do some initial searches to check your search strategy. After this, we recommend that you undertake a full search in this database and then replicate your search in one or more other databases. You will incur duplications, so be alert for this. All databases operate slightly differently but your librarian can help you adjust your search strategy to match them. At master's or undergraduate level, you are unlikely to be looking at unpublished or 'grey' literature unless your supervisor indicates otherwise. You can set up alerts so that should your search identify any new papers, these will automatically be forwarded to you.

Using the databases

Once you have identified the relevant databases, you need to enter the key words and their synonyms (combined appropriately using the Boolean operators AND/OR as discussed above). These will be based on your review question. However, a common error is to search for every word in your question, which is unnecessary. This is because key words often imply the importance of another term; for example, if your review question refers to a topic that is implicitly gendered – for example, 'cervical cancer' – there is no need to search for the term 'women', as this is implied in the initial search term. The key is to identify the most important terms, which, when entered into a database in conjunction with one or two other key terms, will identify research papers that are most relevant to you. Where two terms are likely to identify the same papers, both do not need to be included because you run the risk of excluding papers which do not include reference to both of those terms.

There are two main ways of searching for key terms (+ synonyms). The first is to use 'free text' terms. This is when the key terms are searched for in the text of the paper you retrieve. Alternatively, you might use the terms that have been identified by the database, often referred to as 'controlled headings' or 'Medical Subject Headings' (MeSH). There are advantages and disadvantages to both. For example, if you are searching for an extremely common term, searching as free text is likely to result in an incredibly high number of results. In contrast, if your search term is relatively unusual, you could search the whole text and find no reference at all. Librarians suggest using both ways of searching but your time frame might not allow for this.

Identifying papers for your review

When you review the 'hits' from your database search, you might find that many are not relevant to you – that is, on closer inspection, not all will be relevant to your review question and not all will be research. So, don't panic if you get a long list of 'hits' as many will be irrelevant. You need to go through each of them and check if it is research and whether it meets your inclusion criteria.

If you come across a lot of irrelevant papers, your search might be too broad and you might consider adding another AND string to your search. The alternative is to exclude papers by going through the database. Reading through 1,000 titles can be a relatively quick task if most of the titles can be easily rejected when they are compared with your inclusion criteria. It is often better to have a larger list to work through manually than to limit your search inappropriately using Boolean operators, as discussed above.

Once you have retrieved your results, consider the use of a reference management system such as Endnote or Reference Manager; a variety of systems is available, some of them free of charge. You can use a reference management system to deposit your references, remove duplicates and possibly share with your supervisor. However, this is not essential for a concise review prior to a research study, audit or service evaluation and will likely depend on the technology available via your academic institution.

Refining papers for inclusion

Once you have made an initial review of the papers you have identified, the next stage is to review the abstract of the titles and to compare these against your inclusion and exclusion criteria. Select the papers that clearly address your literature review question, or inclusion criteria. If you are using a reference management database, you can store the reference here. In many cases, the abstract can be included as part of the database entry. The next stage is to obtain the full copy of these papers. You will likely find some papers are not relevant when you see the full paper. You can also undertake 'hand searches' of key journals to identify additional papers. Online databases such as Google Scholar can be used to see how the papers identified have been cited in subsequent papers in order to identify more recent research studies.

There is the possibility you will find a literature review that reflects the focus of your own anticipated review. There is no need to repeat the review but do consider the following questions:

1. Is the review question exactly the same as your question?
2. What is the date of the review? A review that is dated a few years previously will have reviewed papers from at least a year or two before that. This means that your review could focus on the more recent papers. A review that is very current can mean that you do not need to duplicate the work.

If you do identify a recent literature review, consider this a gift – you can structure your own review around this and there is no need to repeat work that has already been undertaken. Do not include any such review as one of your 'research papers' as this might lead to confusion!

Recording your search

Keep an accurate record of your searches: dates of searches, how many titles you identified, how many were relevant, how many duplicates. Many students use a PRISMA flow chart to document their search strategy and results (as documented in Page et al. 2021), if their word count allows. An editable PRISMA statement is available online (https://www.prisma-statement.org/prisma-2020-flow-diagram).

Data extraction/data summary

For someone undertaking a review prior to a small-scale research study, audit or service evaluation, the process of data extraction/data summary is more consolidated than when doing a larger study, but the principles remain the same. Once you have identified the papers that meet the inclusion criteria for your review, you need to 'extract' (or summarise) actual data from the papers that are relevant to your research question. You can do this manually by highlighting or by copying the data (be sure to reference the paper from where it comes) into your notes for further analysis.

Critical appraisal

For a small-scale project, some form of critical appraisal is appropriate. This is usually an informal process; you simply do not have the word count or the time to do an extensive appraisal of each paper. However, you do need to identify which papers are strong and which are not. There are tools available to assist you in the process. For example, both CASP and the Joanna Briggs Institute have critical appraisal tools to match most of the studies that you might come across. The use of a critical appraisal tool is not obligatory but is recommended, as it will provide some consistency in your appraisal and provide evidence of the review process.

Data analysis

At this point, you are ready to start the final stage of analysis. There are different approaches to the analysis of papers in a literature review (see Aveyard et al. 2025) but for those undertaking a small-scale research project, audit or service evaluation, a simple mapping exercise or thematic analysis will be sufficient. A thematic analysis involves identifying the common themes or findings inherent to the research papers included in the review. It is useful to do this in both a summary table and an accompanying narrative analysis. For those of you doing a small-scale research study, the aim of the analysis is to identify what is currently known about your research question and to adjust your research question if necessary, according to the findings of your review. For example, if you find there is already existing literature on your provisional question, this might mean that you can ask a more focused question instead. For someone doing an audit or service evaluation, where the aim of your review is to explore the evidence base for the service you are evaluating, you can include a critique of this evidence base and consider possible strategies if the evidence base is weak.

Final reflection on your review

As you develop and finalise your review, do not be surprised if your overall research question or question guiding your project changes, although this is less likely for those of you undertaking an audit where the question is usually established from the outset. Remember to keep detailed notes on your search strategy as you will need to include these in your final project in addition to how you have appraised and analysed your literature.

Key points

- A separate background and literature review chapter/section is recommended for all projects.
- A literature review question is needed to keep your review structured.
- For small-scale research projects, the focus is on identifying what we already know.
- For audit and service evaluation, the focus is on identifying the current evidence base for the service being evaluated.
- Your review should be proportionate to the size of the project.
- Be as 'systematic' as possible – don't just 'cherry pick' the papers that support your argument.

3

Planning your project

The next step is planning. Once you have settled on a question for your project, which has been shaped by your literature review and background reading, you need to plan your study design. How you shape your study design will be based on a number of factors, including overall practicalities, potential access to participants, availability of participants, and so on. These considerations can be a source of angst and confusion for students and researchers alike, because they can seem to limit what is and isn't possible for your project. They can also influence how your project is perceived, although we would like to point out that there is no such thing as a 'perfect' project and compromises will always need to be made. It is therefore important to ensure that you identify a project that fits the remit for the time and resources that you have available to you and consider the regulations needed to proceed. Thus, reluctance to appreciate the value of all the possible study types we refer to in this book is, we believe, a rather blinkered view. You can learn about research and provide useful data whether you plan to undertake an audit, service evaluation or a small-scale research project – they are all useful projects.

What type of study suits your research question?

In Chapter 1, we introduced the main types of project we include in this book: audit, service evaluation and small-scale research. We advise you to identify which category your project falls into as soon as possible because the type of project you decide to undertake will inform all the decisions you make at the planning stage. How you go about designing your project and the methodological choices you make will be guided by both your study type, which itself is often selected for pragmatic reasons, as well as your philosophical approach.

For example, imagine you are a healthcare student who is interested in the treatment of a condition for a population of patients. You are particularly interested in determining the effectiveness of different drug treatments for this condition. You are aware that the optimum way to do this would be to design a trial in which you compare the treatment effects of two drugs on a group of patients who all have the condition. You would randomise the patients into two groups, administer a different drug to each group, and measure the effects of the drugs on the patients in each group. This study design would likely be a type of randomised controlled trial, otherwise known as a 'clinical trial of an investigational medicinal product' (CTIMP). However, this is clearly way beyond the scope of a small project with a limited time scale and resources. In other words, this is an example of the pragmatic decisions that will affect your choice of study type and its scope. A larger project with a more complex design is something you can consider for your doctoral journey and beyond! Instead, your study should be developed to address a question that is a bit closer to something you have observed in your practice area: in this case, the clinical setting. But it could also be educational in nature or within another organisation, or perhaps even something more personal that inspired your interest in the first place.

If there are guidelines in place for the treatment of a particular condition, you could decide to examine the local records for this patient population to compare the treatments they received with the standards set in the guidelines – this would be a *clinical audit*. Alternatively, you might be interested in whether patients think the treatments they receive for the condition are any good, and you could carry out a survey to assess this. If these are patients who are seen at a local service or clinic, then this would be a *service evaluation*, because you wish to find out whether the service (the treatments they receive) achieves its intended goal. On the other hand, you might want to explore how the condition is treated in a wider population and what the perceptions are of the treatments offered in general. You could design a mixed-methods study inviting volunteers to respond to a survey which you host on a social media site. This would have countrywide coverage and would be considered *small-scale research*.

As we highlighted in Chapter 1, there are more similarities than differences between the different types of project. All three follow a logical process of first identifying a question, which you will then address by collecting either primary data or using secondary sources – data previously collected for another purpose. It is this which will form the essence of your study design: Why this data? How will it answer your question? Is it the most suitable data to answer your question? If it is not the best data for your question, is it the best you can access in the time frame available to you? And how do you intend to go about collecting it? These and other questions are all part of planning your project. We will now go through the steps you need to take to do this, and use examples to illustrate key considerations.

Project planning

You are likely to be accustomed to the processes that will help you plan work schedules or assignments. Planning your research project is, of course, just a particular form of work plan and so the advice we provide at this point will likely be quite familiar to you! Our first recommendation is to start by creating a project outline, sometimes referred to as a protocol document based on the IMRaD structure we introduced in Chapter 1. You can then begin to populate this as you consider the various steps that follow. The golden rules for any project management task are having clear objectives and ensuring frequent communication with other team members. You might not consider yourself as having a 'team' for your project right now, but other people will be involved, which we discuss in Chapter 4. However, at this point we want to remind you of *the* key support for your project, namely your project supervisor.

Supervisor support

If you are undertaking your project as part of the requirements for an educational award – often, but not exclusively, a master's degree – you will have been allocated an academic supervisor. This is someone you will work closely with, and report to, for the duration of the project. For those of you not undertaking research as part of an educational course, we strongly recommend that you identify someone to support you throughout this process, whether that be a clinical supervisor or your manager (or similar), so that you will have someone to bounce ideas off and talk through your intended strategies. For simplicity, we shall refer to this person as your 'supervisor' even if this does not directly reflect their named role or relationship with you.

A supervisor's main role is to listen to your ideas and advise accordingly. They are not in charge of nor will they run the project for you; instead, they act as the 'springboard' or 'consultant' that you need to provide perspective on your ideas. Most supervisors will be allotted a certain time to devote to you, and so it's in your own best interests to use that time wisely and keep in regular touch with them. Remember: early discussions with your supervisor about your study question will help you take the next steps in planning your project (see also the section 'What is my study time frame?' towards the end of this chapter).

Next steps

In the following, we pose questions that you should ask yourself about your study in order to design it and complete your protocol document if required. We will use real-life examples of small-scale research projects, audits and service evaluations. In later chapters, we go deeper and explain how you will carry out the things you have decided to do in your project.

Firming up your research question

At this point you will have established your research question and, as a minimum, carried out an initial search of the literature. If you have not yet decided on your research question, you need to do so as a priority. In theory you need a research question before you can select the method you are going to use. However, this is an iterative process because, as the examples earlier showed, sometimes you will have to adapt your question and project aims based on practical needs. Having discussions with your supervisor will help you with this process.

When you identify your research question, you will also be thinking about what your project outcomes will be. What are you looking to find out? What is it that you hope your study will achieve? This is your overall research aim. Your study objectives are the smaller statements which you use in planning how the overall aim will be met. It is easy to confuse aims and objectives. Your aim and research question are usually interchangeable and guide the whole project. Your objectives are the more focused 'sub-aims' that contribute to your overall aim or question. As mentioned in Chapter 1, the term 'research question' is often used by students, even if their project might technically fall outside what is considered to be 'research'.

Considering the research tradition in which your project sits

In Chapter 1, we discussed the different research traditions, often referred to as paradigms. Identifying where your project sits within the different traditions is important, even if you do not discuss this in detail. The reason why it is important is that you need to ensure your research question and the method you choose to answer it are aligned. An understanding of the research tradition or paradigm will therefore help in deciding how you go about meeting your study aim and objectives – that is, the methods you will use.

Crucially, all research methodologies and methods are underpinned by a philosophical approach to knowledge. This might sound somewhat esoteric – in other words, intended to be understood by a small number of people with this same interest – and you might think that 'philosophy' is too grand a term to use here, but it is important that you understand why you consider the knowledge that you seek will be the most appropriate or valuable for your purposes. Establishing this relates to earlier questions about 'why this data?' and 'how does it answer my question?'

As stated above, the philosophical framework that guides the methodology and methods you might use is usually referred to as a paradigm. For the purposes of study at this level, we recommend that you consider the paradigm and methodology as one – these are the philosophical principles underlying your project. Aside from understanding the basic principles here, we recommend 'light touch' discussion in your final project or thesis. You do not have time to explore the underpinning philosophy in depth but you do need to show the paradigm and methodology are in alignment by identifying appropriate methods. The methods are the particular tools you use to collect and analyse data. You need a clear thread between the overriding paradigm and methodology and methods but it is the methods that you need to attend to in detail.

A paradigm is a worldview that reflects the values and assumptions of the researchers who work within it. For example, beliefs that knowledge can only be certain if derived from observable and quantifiable (measurable) sources is broadly reflective of the *positivist* paradigm; for many years this was the dominant paradigm for the acquisition of all scientific knowledge. As discussed in Chapter 1, this remains an important (but not the only) paradigm through which research is undertaken today. Within this paradigm, the patterns and distributions of phenomena such as health and illness are studied, new drugs are tested, and new treatments are developed that can drastically change the course of a disease, if not eradicate it. Take the COVID-19 pandemic as an example. The vaccines developed for COVID-19, rigorously tested based on the positivist paradigm, are a clear example of this. Because research based on the positivist paradigm relies on the measurement of data, it generally follows that the methodology will employ a *quantitative* design.

An alternative paradigm is *constructivism*, which is based on the assumption that not everything that warrants research can be measured explicitly. Sometimes a more nuanced understanding is required. Take the example of COVID-19 again – our understanding of how people experience a disease might best be achieved by asking their opinion. Together with the researcher, they 'construct' the narrative of their experience, often using words and descriptions to do so, usually employing a *qualitative* design.

From the examples above you can see that a paradigm will provide the framework for designing your project. The most important point is that you show consistency between the paradigm and the methodology and actual methods by which you undertake the study. For example, a study designed to test the effectiveness of a procedure would not be conducted within the constructivist paradigm using qualitative methods. While these two dominant paradigms – positivism and constructivism – are underpinned by completely different philosophies, there is another, 'third' way considered a pragmatism approach. This suggests that there can be different ways of investigating reality according to circumstance, and so a combination of different methods (mixed methods) can be used. Take the example of COVID-19 once more. Remote access to health care during lockdown could be investigated first by surveying (measuring) which patients had used remote access and how, and then by interviewing some of them to explore their experiences in doing so, thus providing a clearer picture of the factors which contributed to the effectiveness (or otherwise) of the service. This is not a means to say 'anything goes' because the justification of pragmatism as a philosophy will need to be convincing. Another warning here is that the data analysis stage of mixed-methods research includes a significant 'integration' step.

If you have chosen to do an audit, then the paradigm you choose is predetermined as positivist (quantitative). Your aim will be to consider whether a phenomenon meets a predetermined published standard. Again, using COVID-19 as our example, all patients admitted to hospital during lockdown should have had a swab on arrival, and had their COVID-19 status recorded. An audit would determine if all patients at your local NHS hospital during a particular period had their COVID-19 status recorded in their patient records (i.e. what percentage and how that compares to the standard set). Service improvement projects such as service evaluations are guided by the universal rationale of evaluating an existing service. While this can be done using methods that sit within different paradigms, in practice many quality improvement projects produce mainly descriptive data as their scope is local. Remember, it is important that you are able to justify your choice of paradigm and methods.

Notwithstanding the advice above, for practical projects such as audit and service evaluation, which are grounded in problem-solving rather than philosophical debate, a discussion of the underlying philosophy might not be relevant: the topic may have been set by a clinician and your task is to undertake the project outlined. How precisely you do this will depend on the requirements of your final project, such as the university's guidance for dissertations; however, it is important to ensure that you are clear about your research question and the way you plan your project. For example, a project that is situated within a positivist paradigm needs to reflect the principles of quantitative data collection and analysis throughout. Likewise, a project that is situated within a constructivist paradigm should stay true to the principles of exploration and understanding throughout. That is to say that whilst you may or may not be expected to articulate the fundamental principles of the paradigm you choose within your final written project, you will be expected to demonstrate an approach to the method of doing your project that is consistent with the underlying philosophical assumptions, whether these are explicit or implicit within your work.

The same principle applies to the concept of research methodologies. There are various definitions of a research methodology, but it is usually understood to be the next layer down from a paradigm and involves the set of practical principles that guide the method for doing a project. For some researchers, the terms qualitative and quantitative constitute methodologies whilst for others, the methodology should be more specific. In this book, we refer to qualitative and quantitative methodologies, as these terms are well embedded in the research literature and probably already familiar to you. Although we recommend that you ensure your paradigm, methodology and method are aligned, we do not think a deep dive into paradigms and methodologies is required at this level of study.

Finally, the depth in which you address the philosophical framework, paradigms or methodology that underpin your study will depend on the requirements of your educational or supporting organisation.

What is the method for your project?

Methods are the tools used to gather and analyse data. The method(s) you decide upon should be guided by your paradigm and methodological approach, not the other way around. For example, deciding to collate and analyse data about student attrition rates for a particular course onto a spreadsheet *without a clear research question*, simply because you have access to these data, is not sufficient. You need to first determine your research question and what sort of data will be appropriate to meet your aims and after that, how you will go about data collection.

Methods for doing research commonly fall into two categories, generally aligning with methodologies: qualitative and quantitative. Whilst this is an over-simplification, it is a useful starting point.

> **Quantitative:** uses numerical data and statistics to answer your research question. Is the answer to your question binary (i.e. yes or no) or easily addressed by numbers or scores? If so, then your methods will collect data that is quantitative in nature.

Take, for example, a *clinical audit* of a maternity unit of 'skin-to-skin contact' between mother and baby after birth. Because this is an audit, the data is numerically measurable – in this case, the proportion of newborn babies who receive skin-to-skin contact within one hour of birth.

A second example would be a *service evaluation* to determine whether the treatments received by patients with rheumatoid arthritis are effective in terms of selected outcomes, including disease activity, pain, biological action and adverse drug reactions. These outcomes can again be measured using quantitative methods.

A final example would be a *small-scale project* using a pre-/post-test design to test a hypothesis – for example, 'patients with back pain who watch a 5-minute instructional video are more likely to continue with prescribed physiotherapy exercises than those who do not'. Ideally this study would be carried out as a 'true experiment' where participants are randomly allocated to a group that receives the instructional video and a group who do not. In reality, this will not be possible for a small-scale project, so an alternative approach is the pre-/post-test design, otherwise known as a 'before-and-after' study. In this type of study, participants are given the instructional video and their adherence to physiotherapy exercises is followed up – but as there is no control group, adherence to physiotherapy exercises among those who did not receive the video cannot be compared. Hence the study is less strong but easier to undertake.

Qualitative: uses words, text, images or documentary sources to answer your research question. In such a study, a binary 'yes or no' answer or a scoring/ranking approach would not suffice.

An example of this would be a *small-scale project* exploring the challenges experienced by nursing students with a physical disability when on practical placement. This project would focus on the feelings, experiences or some other aspect of the students' training that requires words (and not numbers) to capture the essence of their experiences.

Mixed methods: uses a combination of quantitative and qualitative data to answer your study question.

An example of this would be a *service evaluation* investigating the quality of care provided to patients by a particular clinical service via a remote virtual clinic. The data gathered would be a combination of numerical and written answers, as the participants were asked to score various aspects of the service as well as describing what they thought about it.

How will you collect your data?

As outlined in Chapter 1, common data collection methods include interviews (whether individual or group), surveys, questionnaires and documentary analysis. Typically, the method you choose will depend on the type of data you intend to collect. Quantitative data can be gathered via a survey, questionnaire or template/proforma using existing statistics or databases (e.g. healthcare or educational records). Alternatively, data could be based on observation or responses to questions. Qualitative data is usually obtained from interviews, focus groups, descriptive observation, or audio-visual or other documentary material.

Each approach to data collection has its benefits and limitations, which you will need to consider carefully. There is a distinction between prospective (looking forwards) and retrospective (looking back to what has already happened) data collection based on whether the data you intend to collect already exists or not. If data has already been processed but for another purpose, then you can use this data but it will be a secondary analysis. However, data might be newly collected but also termed retrospective, for example, if you plan to ask people to recall their experiences of a particular event.

Prospective data collection means that you capture the data 'live' as events occur in the present moment and perhaps, if you are planning to follow participants or events, into the future. The risk of recall bias is reduced and you can include all data points (variables) that are important for the study. For this reason, it is seen as a very accurate means of data capture. One limitation of this approach is that it is likely to be more time-consuming than retrospective data collection. Another disadvantage is that either you or the participants may alter behaviours to suit the expectations of the study, creating a bias – for example, you could influence the data by selecting the cases to include.

Collecting data retrospectively can be time-efficient because you will be gathering information that has previously been recorded, for example electronic patient medical records or laboratory results, or where the outcomes are already known. A significant limitation, however, is that the quality of data collected will be based entirely on how accurately the information was documented originally, and also whether all aspects of information that you need for your project were recorded. See Ferreira's (2025) reflection on an approach to clinical audit (in Chapter 5), as this illustrates the point very well.

In most countries, strict protocols for data collection assert the right of the individual not to be approached in a way that might seem coercive, and for their information to be held in a manner that is compliant with the law. Absolute compliance from the researcher is needed in this regard and this is discussed in Chapter 4. A detailed discussion of data collection methods is given in Chapter 5.

What is your sampling plan?

Your sampling plan should explain what your sample is, the method of sampling, the sample size and how you will go about obtaining it.

Sampling methods

As you have already identified a research question and undertaken a literature search, you know who your potential participants are – or which things or events are relevant to your study. This is your study population. However, while you will be interested in the whole population – for example, students enrolled on university healthcare degrees in England – it will be unrealistic and impractical to collect data from the entire population. Instead, you need to select a subset or sample from the population to study. If you are undertaking a small-scale quantitative project, you might be able to extrapolate your findings to the population at large. However, in general terms any small-scale project is viewed as a pilot project and its findings preliminary in nature.

There are various methods for obtaining a sample of your population, but how you go about this relates back to the needs of your project. For example, probabilistic/random sampling is where everyone in the population has an equal chance of being invited to participate. For quantitative small-scale research projects, the sampling method will affect the validity of your results. For example, using probabilistic/random sampling for a quantitative study would significantly increase its external validity, meaning a stronger claim to generalisability (the extent to which your results can be applied to other settings). However, for small-scale projects sampling is more likely to be non-probabilistic (e.g. purposive sampling), where you select your sample based on specific criteria. It is important that you understand the approach you take to obtaining your sample and can justify its use.

As a local study (for example, a clinical audit or service evaluation) is clearly based on a particular local population, its findings will not be generalisable. Qualitative methodologies do not seek generalisation of the results to the wider population either, and so do not use probability sampling. However, aiming for greater variability in the sample, by including diversity in participant characteristics, can add to the richness of the study's findings.

Defining the key features of your study population is another important step in deciding who or what can help answer your question, and is therefore reflected in your sample. You do this by setting out the inclusion and exclusion criteria for your project, in a similar manner to that for your literature review. However, now you are declaring what fits or does not fit within the realms of your project. Your inclusion criteria will help identify what your target population is and what characteristics they must possess. The exclusion criteria should not be considered the direct opposite, as it is possible to meet the inclusion criteria yet also possess an attribute that disqualifies inclusion (Patino and Ferreira 2018). So, give careful consideration and balance to your decision, making sure the inclusion criteria are not too narrow, or the exclusion criteria too rigid. For the population of 'students enrolled on university healthcare degrees in England', you might only include students currently attending university and exclude those enrolled but not yet started or those taking time out of study. You might also decide to only include healthcare degrees that lead to a professional qualification. This is all at your discretion but you will need to justify your approach.

Sample size

The size of your sample will again depend on the needs of your project. For qualitative methodologies, the sample size cannot be precisely determined beforehand. There is an argument, though often disputed, that sampling continues until data saturation is achieved: no new insights are to be drawn from the data. So, while your sample size is likely to be small, how small depends on the data you collect. For example, content analysis of free-text answers of a survey will require greater numbers before data saturation is reached than in-depth interviews with participants with a shared experience. This is particularly frustrating for novice researchers because 'what is your sample size?' is a question that is often asked of them by others at the planning stage. What you need to be able to do is provide an estimate and a rationale for this. Taking a pragmatic approach may be appropriate (Denscombe 2021). It can be useful to search for papers and online dissertations for examples of similar designs to yours and identify the approach to sampling. You can also consult your supervisors for guidance.

The best practice for experimental quantitative methodologies is to determine, from the outset, what sample size will be needed (called 'powered') to determine if a true effect exists. A sufficiently large sample size is especially important for hypothesis-testing between groups and for identifying statistical differences. The calculation of sample size will depend on what statistical test you will be using and your study type, for example, pilot studies may be done with smaller samples and you may be able to estimate numbers needed for surveys based on estimates of likely response rates. Whilst this approach is generally beyond the remit of small-scale research projects, it is useful to understand the overriding principles even if these are not relevant due to the size and remit of your project.

A local study still needs a sample large enough that you can show a clear result or are able to answer your research question. A figure of around 50 is considered to be a good starting point for an audit (National Audit Office 2001), but sometimes specialist services do not have as many as 50 cases or service users per year so if this applies to you, then 15 per cent of your overall population is considered to be sufficient. Remember that often the goal is for your clinical leaders or managers to be influenced by the results of your sample, so it needs to be large enough to achieve a suitable, reliable result.

Considerations of equality, diversity and inclusion (EDI)

When planning your project, it is important to consider who your participants will be. For a small-scale research project, it can be tempting to include those who are easiest to reach out to. However, there is a concern that far too much research has been undertaken on 'easily available' populations, meaning the vast majority of people are not represented in research, such as the young, older people and people from minority groups. There have been many initiatives to reduce the impact of this. In the UK, The National Institute for Health and Care Research *Research Inclusion Strategy* (2022) requires that everyone should have the opportunity to participate in research and that researchers should focus on a wider recruitment strategy in order to ensure this is the case. This will help to ensure that research is relevant to everyone in the population, not just select groups, drawing on the principles of social justice. You might want to consider how your project can reach out to a wider range of participants and if this is not possible, reflect on why this is the case.

> **For example,** in the small-scale research project described below, the authors focused on the needs of ethnic minority groups that had not previously been represented in research regarding client needs in follow-up services.

Coughlan et al. (2024) employed the principles of EDI as the focus for their research study, which explored the priorities for follow-up care of participants from ethnic minority groups who had treatment for colorectal cancer with curative intent. Participants in this study were first approached by their clinical teams who, with consent, provided the researchers with the participants' details, including the language they spoke. This enabled the researchers to have the participant information and consent forms translated into the languages required. Non-English language speakers were interviewed via a translator.

Patient and public involvement and engagement (PPIE)

Another consideration when you are generating your question is to consult with members of the public, patients and clients in order to ensure your question, as well as certain aspects of the design of your project, are perceived as relevant by those who might benefit from the study. In the UK, this is usually referred to as patient and public involvement and engagement (PPIE) in research, or service user input. For many small-scale projects, such consultations are possible and probably desirable; even if you do not have the time and resources to undertake a thorough exploration of the views of patients and the general public, understanding the purpose of these consultations is an important part of learning about research. Many university departments have regular meetings with service user groups who invite researchers to discuss their research ideas. If your project is of a fairly general nature, and you anticipate that the views of a pre-established group of people might help to shape your ideas, then gaining access to a group of this kind can be very useful. If your project would be outside the experience of an existing service user group, you might consider seeking advice from patients and the public in a different context. For those of you intending to undertake an audit or service evaluation, then consultation of service users is likely to be of less significance as the importance of the study is implicit in the evaluation of an existing service.

Formulating your research question involves identifying a situation in clinical practice that would benefit from further exploration, in association with a review of existing research and ideally consultation with users of the service you are interested in who can express a view on your research ideas. Once you have identified your research question and whether it fits into the general categories of audit, service evaluation or clinical research, the next step is to determine how you are going to answer it. Consultation with PPIE groups can help you in the design of the method by which the study will be undertaken.

> **For example,** in their small-scale research project to determine the follow-up priorities of colorectal cancer survivors from ethnic minority groups, Coughlan et al. (2024) engaged with members of

a local bowel cancer support group to review the participant information and the study consent form, incorporating the changes suggested to improve readability and accessibility for potential participants.

What is your plan for data collection?

The next step is to determine how you are going to obtain your sample. This might involve recruiting human participants to take part in your study, for example agreeing to complete a questionnaire or to participate in an interview. Or you might decide to extract data from records or databases, but again the details require thought and the correct permissions. Decisions for strategies of recruitment are part of the approvals process, discussed in Chapter 4 and covered in more detail by examples in Chapter 5.

By whatever means you choose to collect your data, it will provide the framework for the results/findings section of your study. The ways in which you store and handle your data are also subject to the relevant permissions, which we discuss in Chapter 4, but it is up to you to plan for this stage. Most data will be recorded electronically, for example on a spreadsheet or simple database. You might see this described as a 'data extraction tool' and give some thought as to the best ways of organising your data. If you are going to perform some statistical calculations, then you will want to record the data in a form that is easy to manipulate – for example, rather than recording 'yes/no' responses, use the binary number system of 0/1.

Importantly you need to consider how you are going to analyse your data. For numerical data it will be by statistical analysis, either descriptive, inferential (correlation, significance and hypothesis-testing) or both. For qualitative data you will need to employ organisation and interpretation to identify patterns and trends (e.g. content analysis, thematic analysis, narrative inquiry or constant comparison methods). Mixed methods also require an extra step of the combination or integration of data types.

The final part of your project planning involves consideration of how the data will be presented to your intended audience. If you are doing a healthcare project you are likely to want your project results to inform clinical practice and perhaps use them as evidence for changing an aspect of practice itself. The nature of a clinical audit is to change or improve practice, so ideally the results, which are usually quantitative in nature, should be kept simple. Descriptive statistics such as pie charts, bar graphs, averages and percentages are often used to explore the results in an accessible but effective way. While complex and technical statistical analysis can be useful, complex analysis is challenging and can pose a problem both for the researcher and the reader. Data analysis and examples will be discussed in more depth in Chapter 6.

What is the time frame of your study?

Developing a timetable will help you to consider key undertakings involved in your study. Do you know what you need and do you have the resources to be able to complete the study on time? Might it be too ambitious? Is it doable in the time frame you have available to you? What about your personal commitments or other academic goals? Creating a timetable or using a scheduling planner will help you keep on track, by detailing what stage you should be at, at any given point in time, particularly if you have fixed deadlines such as assignment hand-in dates. It can be tempting to ignore this step, but it is a tried-and-tested method used by experienced researchers and project managers alike, so give it a go! Being able to visualise milestones for your study is also very useful to support discussions with your project supervisor. A Gantt chart is a very simple example of how you could use a planner, and templates are freely available on the internet. Figures 3.1 and 3.2 are two completed examples of service evaluations, one of a digital triage system in a primary care setting using a Gantt chart (Winser 2025) and the other regarding diabetes also in a primary care setting using a timeline generated using computer software (Michalikova 2026). These set out the master's project over a calendar year, highlighting the important milestones, as well as breaking down the whole project into smaller tasks and detailing when they will begin and end and how long they are anticipated to take. It's likely when working through your ideas that this plan might need to flex and change as your project develops, and that is fine, keep it as a working document that you return to from time to time to help you log your progress and your anticipated actions over your allocated timeline.

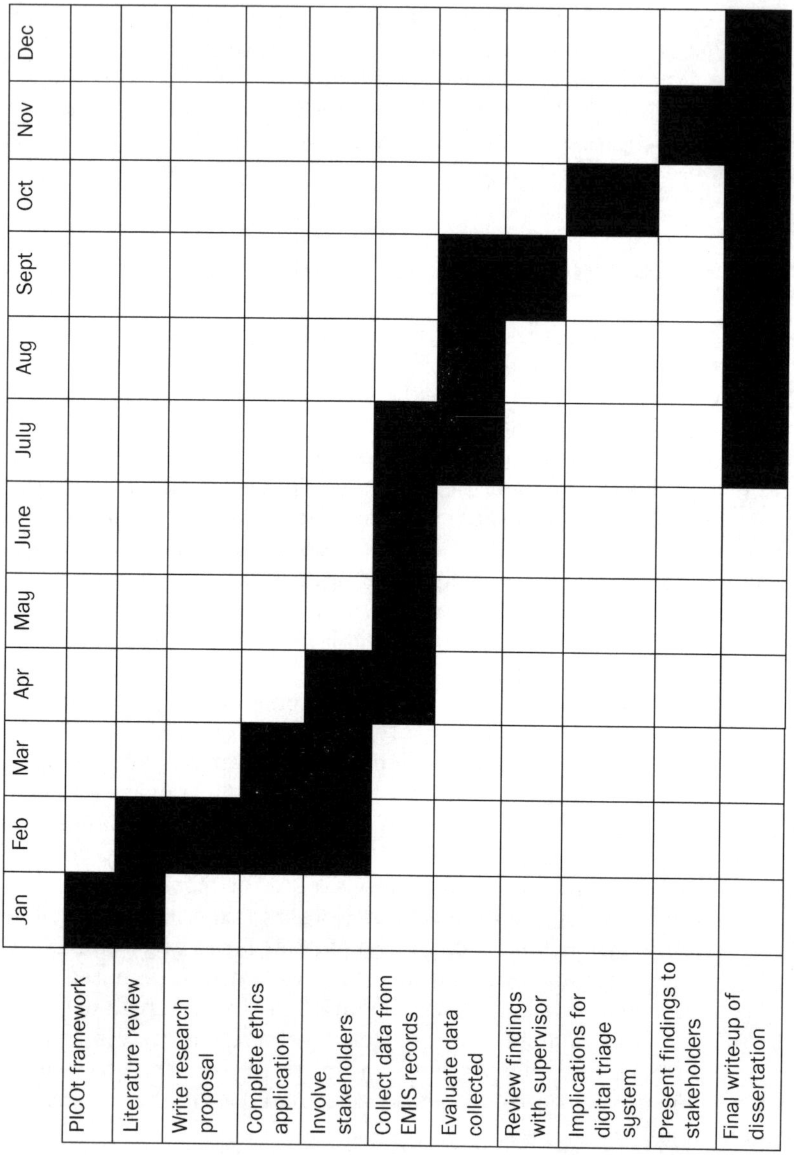

Figure 3.1 Gantt chart for a 'digital triage system' service evaluation project.

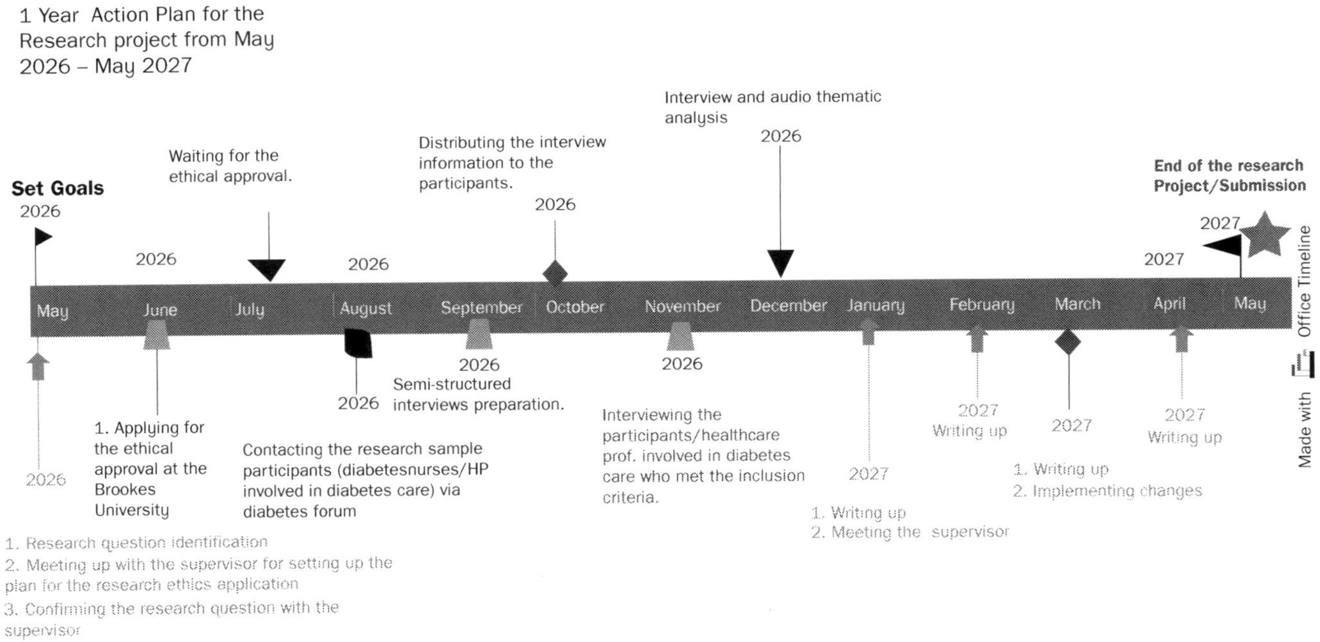

Figure 3.2 Timeline for a 'diabetes care' service evaluation project.

Key points

- Planning your study is key, in the same way that an architect plans the design of a building.
- When you decide on your research question, ensure your methods reflect the philosophical underpinnings of your project.
- It is important to ensure that you get the relevant permissions to conduct your study (see Chapter 4).
- The main focus should be on your method.
- Your project must be small scale – be realistic and pragmatic about what you can achieve.
- Do not rush this stage – it is important to get it right.

4

Ethical approval and other permissions

> **Warning!** This chapter is based on our experience of conducting research in the UK. The processes and actions referred to are therefore based on UK systems and so if you are based elsewhere, you will need to engage with the processes of the country in which you are domiciled. The principles, however, are transferable.

Getting started

At this point in your journey you have formed a question to answer, in addition to your aims, objectives and intended study design: audit, service evaluation or small-scale research project. It is likely you have decided where you want to collect your data, whether this is by investigating patients, clients, students or staff in a clinical or educational setting; examining hospital records, or identifying other sources of information, such as the general public or volunteers. However you intend to gather your data – including if it is to be collected from existing sources – you will need to obtain the agreement of various people in order to proceed. This should be done as early as possible. Some of these agreements will be formal and some informal, which we will discuss later. Failure to obtain the correct permissions can put your project – and ultimately your professional reputation – at risk. It is important to note that as a researcher undertaking a small-scale project, whilst you will be heavily reliant on the cooperation of key individuals, you cannot expect it (Bell et al. 2024): this is why the so-called 'soft skills' of communication and negotiation are vital when you are setting up your project in order to gain access to participants and the potential research site.

It is imperative, therefore, that you discuss your project with all the main players involved in the organisation and development of your project, such as within your university or clinical environment, plus those people who are key within the study setting. These people are generally called 'gatekeepers' because they can grant, or withhold, access to your intended participants and study setting. When you are doing a small-scale project, there are various levels of 'gatekeepers' – some formal, others informal – who provide oversight and ethical scrutiny of your project.

Identifying gatekeepers

Gatekeepers are people who provide permission to access participants and the research site. There are often several official gatekeepers as well as others who should be consulted or kept informed about your project, even if they do not have a formal part to play in its oversight. It's a good idea to spend some time identifying who these individuals are.

In our experience, people are generally very keen to support a small-scale project such as yours. For this reason, you should be confident when you approach them to discuss it. Their goodwill will support you in many ways – before, during and after the project. It is easy to think of some gatekeepers as barriers; they can, and indeed might, create unforeseen obstacles to you undertaking your data collection in the way you want, but more often than not their input will make your project the better for it. They may have some great ideas about the ways things can be done, or open metaphorical doors for data collection. You might find they become valuable later on when you wish to disseminate your findings more widely, and of course they will become part of your network of contacts. They may become colleagues or help guide your future career development. Gatekeepers are vitally important in helping you gather the data you need in the most efficient way. Furthermore, discussions with all interested parties are a matter of professional (and personal) courtesy.

Neglecting to discuss your project with a key contact in your research setting might cause bad feeling. Our advice is that you should consider approaching that key contact as a matter of courtesy, even if you think they won't be interested. In the worst-case scenario, failure to do so could jeopardise your project, but it could also sour relationships between organisations, for example your university and practice partners, meaning it could have an adverse effect on other researchers.

Consider the following story of a student who wished to undertake a service evaluation project (Box 4.1).

Box 4.1: An example of the consequences of missed opportunities to communicate with gatekeepers

A physiotherapy student had been on a practice placement at a newly established clinic, designed for a specific group of people who had suffered traumatic brain injury. The student valued their time at this placement, and for their MSc project wanted to find out more about the users of the clinic and whether it had met their specific needs during their recovery. The student spent time discussing ideas for her project with the physiotherapist who ran the clinic. After discussing the ideas in more detail with her supervisory team, she designed a service evaluation which aimed to collect data via a questionnaire to be distributed to current users of the clinic. The student, supervisory team and clinic staff met to agree the next steps and consider the approvals required for the project. It was established that the project would need some formal approvals (from the university and local NHS Trust) and that the clinic managers and other staff, including medical doctors, would be informed.

The necessary formal approvals were all granted, and the student was ready to start distributing the questionnaires at the clinic and collect data. Unfortunately, the physiotherapist who had been involved changed jobs in the meantime and it transpired had not discussed the project with her managers. When the student went back to the clinic to start her project it resulted in some ill feeling on the part of the clinic manager, who felt she should have known and been consulted. This put the project in jeopardy. The matter was escalated to several other senior staff in the service. Eventually, after clarification and apologies from the supervisory team plus a meeting with senior staff, the project was given the green light.

All of this could have been avoided as a result of better and earlier communication with all the gatekeepers. In the case of this project, they included: the clinic managers, service matron, consultant physiotherapist, governance lead, practice development physiotherapist for students, and head of service.

The first gatekeeper you identify will be your university supervisor if you are a student, or manager if you are an employee. The reason for undertaking your project is likely to be a part of your course requirements, for example as part of a university programme of study, or as part of your employment. In either case, your supervisor or manager will be well aware of your plans, and supportive of them. If you are an independent researcher undertaking empirical research on your own, something increasingly rare nowadays, then you will need the support of key contacts within organisations to help you access data for your project. These key individuals will help you to gain the formal approvals your project will need. We will discuss these processes later.

Ensure that you check with your supervisor or manager who the potential gatekeepers for your project are. In a clinical or educational environment, it is likely there will be a number of individuals who will take an interest in your activities, even if they are not directly involved. A good piece of advice is to inform anyone you identify, even if only out of courtesy. If you are a process-driven person or find management tools useful, you could try using a classic stakeholder matrix to identify the gatekeepers for your project. Using an antenatal clinic as an example, a matrix might look like that in Figure 4.1.

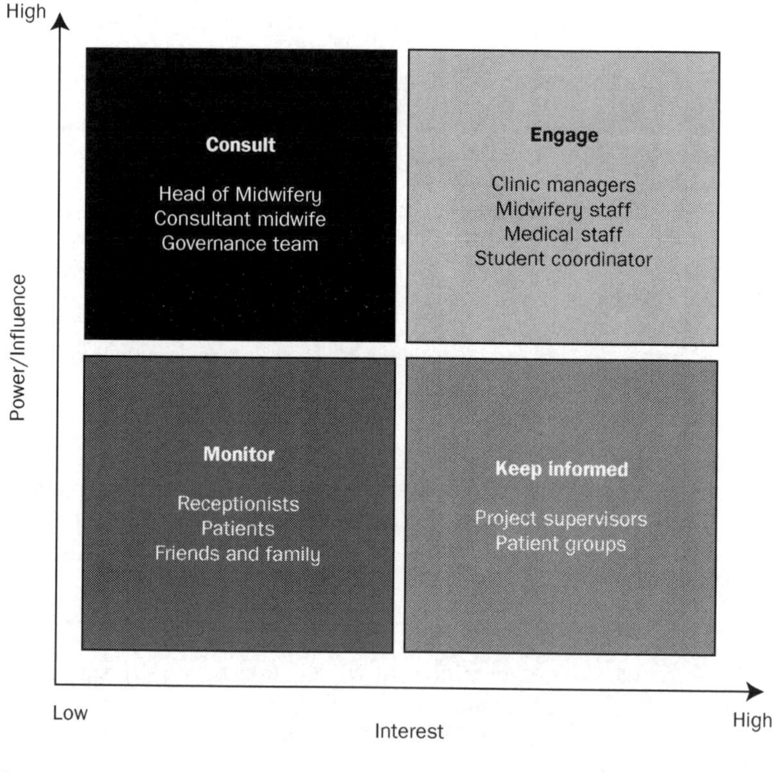

Figure 4.1 Example stakeholder matrix for an antenatal clinic.

Making contact

It goes without saying that your initial contact with a gatekeeper should be professional, polite and quite formal in tone. The most usual method will be by email (see Box 4.2). Take some time to ensure you use correct titles, names and email addresses. Making a good first impression is likely to generate more goodwill towards you and your project, and a similarly courteous response. You can make initial introductions before you have the formal permissions to undertake your project but you must not proceed with any data collection until all those permissions have been obtained.

Box 4.2: Example of initial email to gatekeeper

Head of Social Care

Dear Dr. Brown

I hope this email finds you well.

My name is Jo Bloggs, and I am a master's social work student at Anytown University. I am just about to begin my dissertation which is about the care of asylum-seeking women who have pre-school-age children. My aim is to conduct a service evaluation of the services the women in the local area use, and to interview some social workers to understand their experiences of providing the services on offer.

I will seek ethical approval from my university and will register my project as a service evaluation with the governance team within the service. Having had some informal chats with several of my practice supervisors, there is interest in my study.

The purpose of this email is to request your agreement for me to conduct my research via the social work services. The project will take place from October 2026 to March 2027. I will be inviting social workers (both qualified and those in support roles) to be interviewed but will not disrupt any normal activities. Naturally, I will be pleased to share the findings of my dissertation with you and the rest of the team when completed.

If you are willing to agree to this request, please can you reply to this email, as it will support my research application.

Many thanks in advance,

Jo Bloggs

What will gatekeepers need to know?

Whilst some key gatekeepers, such as your project supervisor or manager, will be intimately involved in the development of your project proposal and will already know about it in detail, other people you wish to keep informed or get an informal 'go-ahead' from, are unlikely to know much about your project; they may not even know who you are. You will probably want to prepare a summary or brief outline of your project for them. This will of course include the title, purpose, aim and design. It is important you use 'lay language' and emphasise the importance and relevance of the project, and introduce both yourself and your supervisor. You need to show you are credible, and that you have – or will get – the appropriate permissions to do your project. They are likely to be interested in the practical details of how your project might affect them. For example, will it impact staff members? Will it inconvenience anyone? How long will it take? Will it cost money? Will it provide useful information?

Having a short plain language summary of your project available to attach to emails or letters of introduction is a good idea. We emphasise the word 'short' because it is important to be succinct in getting your message across to people whose time is important. Practise explaining your project in a few sentences so that if you are introduced to one of your gatekeepers, or if you are invited to describe your project in a meeting, you can do so both confidently and succinctly. This summary can be used or adapted when obtaining subsequent permissions such as ethical approval. In the example above, the student might also prepare a plain language summary document including more details, such as that shown in Box 4.3 (adapted from Pugh 2023).

Box 4.3: Example summary project details

Title: Care Provision for Women with Pre-school-age Children in Anytown Trust

Aim: Asking how social workers navigate providing their care service to women who are seeking asylum who have pre-school-age children.

Rationale: (1) There is little national guidance, (2) numbers are rising locally as newly designated dispersal area, (3) wish to compare to service standards.

Design: Qualitative, semi-structured interviews. Up to 5 social workers invited to participate.

Data/confidentiality: Anonymity of interviewees assured, no personal data.

Outcomes: Perceptions and strategies employed by social workers to provide person-centred care as they gain experience in providing services for women with pre-school-age children and who are seeking asylum; explore the support needs of social workers in providing this service.

Inclusion: Social workers who provide care for women with pre-school-age children seeking asylum within their caseloads.

Governance – oversight of your project and obtaining formal permissions

So far, we have discussed the 'local' or 'informal' permissions you will need in order to undertake your project and indeed to assess whether your project is feasible. You will have noticed that the student in the example above had already indicated they would require some more 'formal permissions' to conduct their study, beyond agreeing it with the various local gatekeepers. Formal permissions need to be obtained from people who have official regulatory responsibilities within the organisations potentially involved in your study – your organisation/employer and the organisation where you intend to collect data.

Permission from your sponsor

Your sponsor will be your university or employer and it is they who will take overall responsibility. Should anyone come to harm or should data be used inappropriately, your university/employer will ultimately be accountable. Although such incidents are rare, it is important to be aware of who is accountable and why governance procedures are put in place. You may find your organisation referred to as your 'project sponsor' or something similar. In practical terms, this means that the organisation will provide resources to support your project, usually in the form of administrative and structural support, but it could also be financial in some cases. It is usually understood that the sponsor takes legal responsibility for the project, and it is for this reason that your sponsor needs to know everything about your project. They will ensure that the project supports the organisation's mission and that it is conducted according to relevant regulations and standards of good research practice.

Each organisation will have its own systems in place, and so it is important that you become familiar with the processes within your own organisation and that you adhere to them. The support offered by the sponsor will include resources, such as people to help navigate you through this step. Luckily, as your project will be 'small' in nature (which is possibly why you are reading this book), this shouldn't be particularly onerous.

Each organisation will require you to submit an application to conduct your research, where you show how you have planned your project, and address any ethical and governance issues which might be required by the organisation (see Box 4.4 below). You might consider this application to conduct your research as a formal permission, built on the groundwork of the informal permissions discussed earlier. You may hear people talk about 'getting ethics'. In fact, the formal permissions required are broader than ethics, although the permissions needed for your study will include ethical approval. Your sponsor will require you to meet the standards of local ethics boards, in addition to any other wider ethical approval. In short, the institution through which you are undertaking your project will require that all permissions are obtained. It is only when your sponsor (i.e. your institution) is satisfied that you have done this, will they agree to take overall responsibility for your project.

Permission from an ethics board

For some projects, further ethical approval might be needed. Often, low-risk projects and those not categorised as 'research', such as audit or service evaluation, do not require external ethical approval but do need some further approvals, and your sponsor will confirm what these are (see below, p. 66). With your sponsor's agreement secured, you need to consider any further approvals required, such as from a local Research Ethics Committee (REC) or an equivalent. This means an ethics board that sits outside your sponsor or organisation. For a project involving staff and students within an educational establishment, you are unlikely to require permissions beyond those of your sponsor and local university. However, for projects involving staff or patients within the hospital setting, further permissions will probably be needed. These will vary from country to country and will require varying amounts of documentation; however, the documents needed will usually mirror those already prepared for local ethical considerations and sponsorship. See Box 4.4, which lists the information required to complete an approval application.

Box 4.4: Core elements to consider (for *all* approval applications – both sponsorship and ethical approval)

Study title – sets the scene and should ideally convey what the study is about (and give an idea of methodology).

Introduction/background – this is the overview, where the research problem, and so justification for the study, is made clear. You may add a rationale here to show what your study will add to existing knowledge. Why the research question is worth asking or why it is worthwhile to participants or the wider service delivery.

Study aim – what you intend your research to achieve, and your objectives (smaller parts that make up the overall aim).

Study design, methods of data collection and data analysis – a design and approach (methodology) should be used that reflects the aim and objectives of the study. Methods of data collection and data analysis. Study time frames.

Study setting, population/sample – definition of the study population/sample, including sample size, and an explanation of where and how data will be collected. Description of eligibility – i.e. inclusion and exclusion criteria.

Recruitment and consent – how participants are identified and recruited. Here the process of gaining informed consent is detailed as is use of documents, such as participant information sheets, consent forms and recruitment posters.

Ethical and regulatory considerations – this is where you detail how your study will be managed to uphold the principles we introduce below, in particular any risk/benefits to participants and how the data collection methods ensure participant dignity, and confidentiality and data security are upheld. Compliance with necessary authorities and gatekeepers is part of this.

Other elements might include an independent review of the study, patient and public involvement, estimates of timings and costs, and plans for outputs and dissemination after study completion.

Supporting documents might include participant information, consent forms, confirmation emails from gatekeepers, study flow charts, resource plans, recruitment posters or social media wording.

The process of gaining permissions to undertake your project requires much thought and attention, so it is important to be as efficient as possible. Try not to feel daunted, take each process step by step, and act promptly on each email or instruction in order to reach the data collection stage of your project, which is your goal! Also remember that there are plenty of resources available to help you do this, available either from your sponsoring institution or other public institution.

The information for your project can be summarised as certain core elements. You may notice that these are similar to those generally required in a project protocol, something you may already have written.

The overall purpose of the documentation you provide to gain research approvals will be: to describe what you want to study, how you intend to do it, whether it is worth doing, what the risks are to participants, and how these will be minimised or managed. Importantly, you will need to show you have considered the essential issues of project governance (meaning you have identified the main project processes plus the roles and responsibilities of those involved) and protected the wellbeing of any research participants. You want to show that you are competent to do your project within the resources and time frame you have available to you. You will also need to demonstrate that you have adhered to ethical principles. It might be the case that there are several rounds of correspondence between you and the sponsor or committee representatives before final approval is given. This is another reason it pays to start early. Most people find that although this can be frustrating at times and may include several revisions, the final product (which is essentially your study plan) will be far better for it.

Ethical principles that apply to audit, service evaluation and small-scale research

The principles that guide the ethical conduct of research are addressed in many documents, including the Belmont Report (1979) and the Declaration of Helsinki; the latter is updated regularly to reflect current practices and perspectives pertaining to research ethics. Adherence to an ethical framework when you consider the potential ethical issues that are relevant to your project will be useful, as you can then be reasonably confident that you have addressed the key points. There are many ethical frameworks available. In this book, we refer to the four principles cited by Beauchamp and Childress (1994), a framework which has remained popular over time and is frequently referred to by scholars and researchers worldwide. The four principles are: justice, autonomy, beneficence and nonmaleficence. Let us explore each of these in turn.

Justice refers to the overriding consideration of fairness in the delivery of a project. Embracing equality, diversity and inclusion (EDI) is one step towards promoting the principle of justice. Doing so will mean that research is made available to people outside the majority group, thus ensuring that everyone's voice is heard.

Autonomy refers to the right of the individual to choose whether to participate in your project and their right to withdraw at any time. This requires careful consideration on your part of the way in which you introduce the project to potential participants to obtain their informed consent. This does not involve providing appropriate information but also ensuring that participants have the capacity to understand that information and are not being put under pressure from colleagues or family to participate. You will be required to write a clear summary of your project in 'lay language' to potential participants. These 'participant information sheets' ought to provide as much information about the study as possible, including the risks and potential benefits to taking part. This is why this is such an important part of the process.

The principle of autonomy also protects the right of the individual to refuse to consent to take part and their right to be protected from any pressure or coercion from anyone who might encourage them to do so. We refer to this in subsequent examples where participants have an ongoing relationship with the researcher and might then feel 'obliged' to take part. If you feel that this might be the case, there are various steps you can take to limit this, and your supervisor will discuss how this might be done. For example, Maddison (2023) provides a clear recruitment strategy for researchers to avoid recruiting students into a project for whom they have direct responsibility.

Until fairly recently, the principles of informed consent and the need for explicit consent prior to research resulted in few studies being undertaken with individuals who lack capacity but this has changed in recent years due to recognition of the importance of research to understand the needs of those who cannot consent. Legal principles vary in different countries. In the UK, no one can consent on behalf of an individual who lacks capacity (with the exception of someone who has a lasting power of attorney) and so next-of-kin cannot be asked to provide consent. However, they might and should be asked for their views about participation. Instead, the requirement for consent to participation in an audit, service evaluation or small research project is waived in the same way as consent prior to a clinical procedure – participation is generally considered acceptable if the study entails only minimal risk and hence is 'not against' the best interests of the participant. O'Shea et al. (2025) provide a detailed account of considerations to be made when potential participants have dementia. For those who cannot consent and who lack the capacity to do so, participation in research is more complex since additional reassurance is needed that it is appropriate for them to do so.

Nonmaleficence is the duty to do no harm. Harm includes any act that might compromise the safety or dignity of the participant. This includes the digital safety of the participant and assurance that their privacy will be respected. Some projects involve more risk than others. For those of you undertaking a small-scale project such as the ones we refer to in this book, the risks are usually minimal but it is important to recognise what these might be. Interviews, for example, might trigger unpleasant or upsetting memories, even if fleetingly. However, this is likely to be a consideration rather than a red flag to undertaking the project overall. This is because research in this area has found that whilst discussion of very sensitive topics might lead to distress, this distress is usually transient and afterwards participants report being glad they took part. This was the experience of McCallum (2022), for instance, who interviewed recently bereaved individuals whose relative had died in the emergency department. And although a questionnaire might be burdensome to complete and it might also trigger unpleasant emotions, it gives participants an opportunity to air their views. There are, of course, instances where the intervention proposed might lead to harm or serious side effects. The Northwick Park phase 1 critical trial is an example of this, in which six paid participants who were invited to take part in a study that involved the administration of a new drug with unknown side effects had a severe reaction (Dixon 2006). This was a clear violation of the principle of nonmaleficence.

Beneficence is the duty to do good. Every project, be it an audit, service evaluation or small-scale research study, aims to promote the good of future patients, clients, colleagues and/or students. However, in recent years there has been increasing emphasis that research and small-scale projects can benefit the people who take part. This is sometimes referred to as the 'research effect'. The reasons for this are diverse but include the opportunity to interact with similar others involved in the project, the opportunity to reflect on previous experiences with a researcher or project leader, or the simple fact of 'feeling heard'. Many participants also report feeling altruistic having taken part (Carrera et al. 2018). So, whilst traditionally researchers were encouraged to state clearly in a letter of invitation to participate in research that there would be limited benefits to doing so, this emphasis has now changed to reflect the known benefits of participation.

When you are preparing your ethics permission documentation, we recommend that you use the four principles as an aide-mémoire or lens through which to consider the risks inherent in your project and how you will mitigate against them. It is important to state in the documentation what precautions you will put in place to mitigate against the risks you have identified, even if you consider them minor. One way to do so is to identify existing studies that have undertaken a similar method to you and see how they went about it, which you can then reference in your own documentation. This is not to say that every approach you read about will be an example of good practice, but it will provide some evidence of what has been previously approved. Some authors document issues encountered in a project, and you might get tips and hints from relevant papers about the methods used.

Further to this idea is to make reference in your ethical approval documents to research that has looked at the potential for harm to participants in different contexts. For example, having received ethical approval, Lascelles (2024) explored the experiences and support needs of adult family members, partners and friends who care for adults at risk of suicide using an online questionnaire. She included an additional questionnaire in order to assess any harm resulting from the carers' participation in the research process. Responses indicated a clear willingness to participate and no indication that completion of the questionnaire resulted in any harm. Making reference to studies such as these can be included in your permissions application as evidence that you have carefully considered your approach and identified that the risks to your participants are minimal. See Box 4.5 for guidance on the main principles of good research practice.

Box 4.5: The main principles of good research practice

There is a wealth of advice for researchers regarding the various ethical and statutory principles and frameworks for conducting research, such as guidance from regulatory and professional bodies and institutions. Key resources include:

The concordat to support research integrity – a national policy statement for good research conduct developed by UK universities, research institutes and others undertaking research (https://www.universitiesuk.ac.uk/what-we-do/policy-and-research/publications/concordat-support-research-integrity).

The UK Research Integrity Office Code of Practice for Research – promotes good practice and how to prevent misconduct (https://ukrio.org/ukrio-resources/publications/code-of-practice-for-research/) – and the Recommended Checklist for Researchers (https://ukrio.org/ukrio-resources/publications/code-of-practice-for-research/).

For health research in particular, the Medical Research Council's Principles and Guidelines for Good Research Practice (https://www.ukri.org/publications/principles-and-guidelines-for-good-research-practice/) and the International Conference on Harmonisation Good Clinical Practice principles (ICH GCP), which are founded on the ethical principles of research enshrined by the Declaration of Helsinki following the Second World War (www.ichgcp.net).

The main ethical principles you should consider in your application are the dignity, rights, safety and wellbeing of your participants. For a small empirical project such as yours, while you may consider it unlikely that there are any ethical risks, maintaining overall excellence and integrity at all stages of your project is imperative. So, emphasise that you have given thought to the following, which are based on the three unifying principles of the Belmont Report (1979): How will you (as far as you can) protect them from any risk of harm? This is the principle of nonmaleficence or 'do no harm'. What information do they need to know beforehand? If you are interviewing people, for example, is it possible they may become upset? What can you do to support them (and yourself) if this happens? How can you protect their sensitive information, for example by ensuring confidentiality and anonymity? Who will have access to the data and how will you protect and store it? In the UK this is governed by the General Data Protection Regulation (GDPR) and the UK Data Protection Act 2018.

Show respect for the autonomy of potential participants by seeking their informed consent to take part in (or contribute data to) the study. Will you provide an information sheet telling participants what to expect and what the study involves? Will you ask for written confirmation of their consent to participate? How will you make it clear they are not obliged to take part, and what would happen if they changed their mind?

Finally, demonstrate the principle of justice by showing that any research procedures are fair and non-exploitative for all. For example, is it reasonable to ask your participants to travel to meet you for a focus group without offering them travel expenses?

Ethics approval: where to apply

Where you apply for approval from a research ethics committee will likely depend on your sponsoring organisation, but also on where you are conducting your research. If you are a university student or employee, then you will need to apply to your university/employer directly for their ethical approval. This is invariably the first application you need to make to gain ethical approval for your study. For some low-risk projects, this may be sufficient, especially if your recruitment and data collection methods are external to the National Health Service (NHS). This means that your whole project must lie outside the remit of the NHS, including recruitment; in such cases, recruitment strategies using social media are possible.

However, and again in the UK, if your study involves NHS facilities, staff or patients/service users, then you may additionally need to apply to an NHS ethics committee. This process is managed by the Health Research Authority (www.HRA.NHS.UK) using a web-based system called the Integrated Research Application System (IRAS). Importantly, this only applies to certain projects: those which are understood by the HRA to be of higher risk (e.g. experimental designs, interventions or invasive designs, such as projects that require tissue samples to be taken). Regulations around which research studies require further scrutiny by the Health Research Authority are subject to change and will be different in countries other than the UK.

As mentioned earlier, audit and service evaluation generally do not fall under the remit of the HRA. Often, but not always, these projects do not involve the collection of new data, have a local context and are not generalisable. Audits, service evaluations and other small-scale projects will require local approval, but this application process is not to the NHS REC or via IRAS (see section below). Some of course might be viewed as research according to other definitions. When undertaking a project involving the NHS, it is therefore vital to establish right at the outset if your project is considered research. You do this by using the HRA decision tool (https://www.hra-decisiontools.org.uk/research/redirect.html).

It's important here to note that many peer-reviewed health journals do not publish research papers reporting audits or service evaluations without ethical approval, although professional journals that are more practice focused such as the *Nursing Times* and *British Journal of Midwifery* may do so. If getting a paper published in a peer-reviewed journal is an important goal, then you need to be aware of this.

Once you have obtained the appropriate ethical approval, some organisations require further formal approval for you to undertake data collection. For example, in the UK, projects undertaken within the NHS also need to obtain what is currently referred to as 'Capacity and Capability' approval to collect data from each NHS site you wish to visit. This can take extra time. If you are not a member of NHS staff or a healthcare student on placement, you will additionally need to apply for a research passport. This mechanism enables you to obtain an Honorary Research Contract or Letter of Access to carry out your research within the NHS. Again, this can be a frustratingly slow experience at some NHS Trusts.

Non-NHS organisations such as local authorities, councils and third-sector organisations will have their own approval processes, although not necessarily a formal ethics committee. Of course, you will still need to seek permission via their own processes if this applies to your project. The Social Care Institute for Excellence has a research ethics committee, but does not review student projects. Instead, such applications require completion of a form for this purpose. Occasionally you and your project supervisor may also be asked to attend a meeting.

As you can see, the processes for obtaining both ethical approval and organisational approval can be time-consuming. We advise that you identify the approvals you need at the planning stage of your project and adapt as necessary if the time frame available to you does not allow for this.

Audits, service evaluations and other healthcare projects

For those of you undertaking an NHS project (involving NHS premises, staff or data), which, as described above, is not classified as research by the Health Research Authority (HRA) in the UK, you will need to seek approval locally from the healthcare setting where the data is to be collected. As with other approvals, each institution will have its own processes and forms for this purpose. Remember, you will still require the approval of your sponsor.

For example, at our local NHS Trust the approvals process for non-research empirical projects involves registering the study on a central system overseen by clinical governance teams. Projects must fulfil certain criteria to be approved, which include having a named supervisor who is a clinical staff member with project oversight, who is responsibile for the management and completion of the study. Also required is a description of the project aims, objectives, outcome measures, methodology and time frames. As we saw in Chapter 3, audits involve collecting data about an aspect of care that can be compared to a set of predetermined, recognised or pre-established standards, while service evaluations involve collecting data from service users to assess a particular service. Although the registration form is far simpler and shorter to complete for these two study types, the main elements that we introduced as being key for ethical approval are still relevant here. Responsible individuals in a clinical governance role can accept or reject the application for a local project to be carried out and will need to be satisfied that the study is worthwhile and poses no risk (including financial) to the organisation.

Box 4.6: Example of a local service evaluation application to an NHS Trust

Title: Service Evaluation of Intrauterine Contraception Service at Named Hospital

Description: This project seeks to evaluate the service experience of women receiving contraception of an Intrauterine Contraceptive Device/System (IUD/IUS)

1. Aspects of care the project seeks to improve

Since the commencement of this service in 2023, no service evaluation has examined if the current offering meets women's needs.

2. The criteria that are being audited.

Service users advised 6-week follow-up care by the GP or earlier if needed, but to date this has not been evaluated.

3. The standard for each criterion.

Overall satisfaction with their contraception (IUD/IUS), numbers of contraception failures (unplanned pregnancy), numbers following advice given (checking placement of IUD/IUS), numbers accessing follow-up at 6 weeks, assess problems identified.

Methodology: Retrospective survey design of women who received any form of IUCD at said clinic since the service began (previous 3 years).

Records will be screened to identify relevant patients, excluding any deceased or individuals opting out of research contact. This cohort will be contacted first by letter from the clinical lead consultant of the service notifying them of the audit and inviting completion of an online questionnaire. Completion of the survey requires confirmation of consent. Non-responders will also receive an email or telephone call to complete the survey.

The costs of postage will be met externally. No personal data is used outside of the hospital. Anonymised pooled data and survey findings will be stored safely according to data protection principles and used to complete the dissertation project.

This service evaluation is for fulfilment of an MSc degree by a student (i.e. who has current practice placement status, including access to patient records). Supervised by [named individual and credentials], with agreement/oversight of the service [named consultant].

Service evaluations are encouraged by the HRA as fulfilling criteria for standalone MSc projects.

The findings of this project may also be used by the local team as part of ongoing service improvement.

Dates: Start and completion dates.

Manager's comments: Named University will also undertake an approval/governance process for individual undertaking of this local project.

Box 4.7: Example of a local audit application to an NHS Trust

Title: Audit to Assess Compliance with Completion of VTE Assessment in Maternity and Accuracy of Assessments and Thromboprophylaxis Prescriptions

Description: Ensuring timely and accurate VTE assessment and correct thromboprophylaxis prescription are meeting local standards for VTE prevention.

Methodology: Audit (of past 6 months) to assess if:

1. A VTE assessment has been completed at booking, 28 weeks' gestation (if relevant) and current admission/postnatally.
2. That VTE assessment is accurate and consistent on two local electronic record systems.
3. Weight is being documented and most recent weight is being used for thromboprophylaxis prescription.
4. If the correct recommendation is being followed, i.e. correct prescription.

N.B. We would aim for a standard of >95% for each criterion.

Dates: Start and completion dates.

Manager's comments: Named University will also undertake an approval/governance process for individual undertaking of this local project.

Once you have the necessary permissions

There are plenty of other things that you can be doing while you are waiting to receive confirmation that you can start your project, so use your time wisely. You cannot (and must not) start any recruitment or data collection until all your approvals are in place, but you can usefully spend time on some further preparation. This will include administrative tasks like organising the copying of leaflets, formatting your data collection instrument (e.g. a spreadsheet) and addressing logistical questions, such as how to get to an unfamiliar setting or where you can store your equipment and belongings. You might consider asking your gatekeepers if you can briefly introduce your project to their teams at a meeting or other forum. If you decide to do this, a valuable exercise is to plan and practise delivering a short introduction to your study, covering what you want to find out and how staff might be able to help you. And make sure you give a good impression of yourself and your study. Even if you don't need anything from them, it's important that they know who you are and why you might be present in their space! Not being a stranger will make being 'in the field' much more comfortable.

You also need to complete your literature review. When you start your project, it is easy to get caught up in the immediacy of data collection. You may sometimes forget the obligations you have to your sponsor, and that they remain a resource for you. Naturally, you will remain in regular contact with your project supervisor, but the other individuals you contacted as part of your application can also provide advice and support throughout the life cycle of your study should issues arise, as unfortunately they may well do. Such issues include finding that recruitment of participants to the study is taking much longer than you expected, or that your data is incomplete and you need to amend what is collected and change your study timelines.

At project completion

A final reminder here is to fulfil your obligations to your study sponsor and other gatekeepers by notifying them when your study has been completed. Local systems will likely require records to be kept of projects that have been completed, and on what date. You can save yourself, and others, the hassle of being chased for this information by letting them know what they require in a timely fashion. We are hopeful that you will be communicating the findings of your project far and wide, and this is a part of that process (see Chapter 7). And, of course, remember to thank everyone who has supported you and your study throughout its various stages.

Key points

- Permissions needed for a project are both informal and formal – your project will not get off the ground without both!
- All projects need ethical and organisational approval from your sponsor – usually your educational institution or employer.
- If your project is undertaken in a different institution, you need to check the permissions required – for example, further ethical approval from an external research ethics committee together with formal organisational permission.
- Ensure that you are able to obtain these permissions in the time available to you.

5

Methods of data collection

In Chapter 3, we discussed the importance of planning your project and in Chapter 4 we explained what permissions you need to carry it out. So, at this point you have identified your question and know how you intend to answer it, including your overall approach. In this chapter, we explore in detail the methods for collecting your data. We will provide examples both from students and the published literature that illustrate the different methods of data collection for the three types of project we discuss in this book: audits, service evaluations and small-scale research projects. It is important to note that none of the methods are specific to any particular type of project – each can be used in a variety of projects. Furthermore, it is possible to combine the methods of data collection, known as mixed methods. As most of the methods of data collection you will use are well established and in widespread use, we will signpost you to key texts. In this chapter, we will discuss:

1. **Data collected from patient records or other documents:** This data already exists and so its collection might seem relatively straightforward, but not only will you need to be careful to identify the permissions required (see Chapter 4), you also need to navigate how the data is organised or formatted as it is unlikely to be arranged perfectly to suit your purposes. Those undertaking an audit or small-scale research project often use existing records from various sources as data for their project, combining this with another approach in a mixed-methods design.

2. **Data collected via questionnaires/surveys:** This is where you collect data in an organised way, for example from patients, clients, carers, colleagues or students. Most of you will be familiar with being asked to complete a survey or questionnaire, maybe as part of market research or after purchasing an item. These are not as simple to construct or design to achieve meaningful responses as might be imagined. When undertaking an audit, service evaluation or small-scale research project, questionnaires/surveys are often used as the method of data collection.
3. **Data collected via individual or group interviews:** This is where you collect data in a less structured format. This method of data collection usually delves deeper and with more complexity than when using a survey or questionnaire. Obtaining data using individual or group interviews is highly dependent on the skill of the researcher conducting the interviews. This is not a method you are likely to use if you are undertaking an audit, but you could do so if conducting a service evaluation or small-scale research project.

As discussed in Chapters 1 and 3, the method of data collection needs to be appropriate for your overall research/project question, after consideration of the philosophical framework or paradigm in which your project sits. What follows are examples of projects using different methods of data collection together with discussion of their various attributes.

Throughout this book, we emphasise that all of the various data collection methods can usually be used in an audit, service evaluation or small-scale research. There are some methods, however, that fit different projects better than others – for example, if you are going to conduct an audit, you are likely to choose quantitative methods or data extracted from some form of documentation. This is because the audit needs to focus on clear outcomes which are measurable numerically. For service evaluations and small-scale research projects, each of the various methods of data collection is frequently adopted.

Data collected from patient records or other documents

There are lots of data that are already in existence and which you might be able to utilise for your project, such as patient records, guidelines for the management of a particular condition, or educational handbooks which illustrate how courses are delivered. Reviews of records, sometimes known as chart reviews, or other documentation are attractive because the data already exists; it just needs to be extracted after gaining the appropriate permissions. This method is not restricted to audit where it is used for quality improvement purposes; it can also be used for a small-scale research project where the aim is generalisation of the findings. For example, Oozageer Gunowa et al. (2021) used existing available documentation from five higher education institutions to identify how educators incorporate principles of equality, diversity and inclusion within their teaching.

In all circumstances you will need to engage with the organisations with which you wish to work and apply for the necessary permissions (see Chapter 4). Whilst audit is an accepted mechanism for quality improvement within the UK, and there are procedures in place for accessing patient notes for example, some organisations (e.g. educational establishments) might be reluctant to release any documents for external scrutiny, even for the purposes of research, and are under no obligation to do so.

Existing data is most often used for audit; however, it can also be used in a service evaluation or other small-scale research project. A larger project might employ mixed methods, using existing data from patient or student records as part of the overall design.

The example we use of a project using pre-existing data is from an audit of hospital patient records undertaken by Ferreira (2025) for a master's degree project (see Box 5.1). The outcome of interest – the management of acute otitis externa – was recorded in patient medical records. The information required could be extracted from the patient records and then compared with the pre-determined, national standard for the management of the condition. To do this, an appropriate sample of records would be necessary. However, achieving this is not as straightforward as it sounds; the way members of staff use systems and attend to their record-keeping varies and consequently the completeness and quality of the data that is found in these existing sources may prove to be of a poorer standard than expected, thus limiting the quality of the audit. It is unlikely that you will be able to 'fill in the gaps' where there is missing data, unless you are able to extract it from another source, or seek clarity from the data originator. For this audit the senior nurse in the ear, nose and throat (ENT) centre wanted to determine whether the national standard (NICE 2024) for treating otitis externa (an infection of the outer ear) was being adhered to in the local setting.

Box 5.1: Example of a project in which data was collected from patient records

Title: A Clinical Audit of the Management of Acute Otitis Externa in an Ear, Nose and Throat Centre at an NHS Trust Hospital in England.

Background: In the specialist ear, nose and throat (ENT) department, the management of patients with otitis externa (OE) had been noted to vary among the clinicians treating the condition. The available NICE guideline (2024) around the management of OE recommends:

1. Cleaning the external ear canal from debris with micro suction and providing a 7- to 14-day course of topical antibiotics ear drops with or without topical steroids.
2. Taking an ear swab for microbiology cultures in all cases of treatment failure, chronic OE and in patients that are immunocompromised or at high risk of severe infection.
3. Providing a follow-up if symptoms are not improving after 48 hours, are not resolved after 2 weeks and for immunocompromised patients.

Aim: To conduct a clinical audit to determine if ENT clinicians in the local department were compliant with the NICE guideline (2024) in the management of OE and understand the implications of current practice on treatment outcomes. The results of this clinical audit could determine whether the current care provided is optimal or, alternatively, inform areas for improvement that could lead to better quality of care.

Method: A retrospective clinical audit was conducted reviewing the records of 144 patients diagnosed with acute OE over a 5-month period. Data extracted from electronic patient records (EPRs) and the GP referral unit electronic patient database were compared against NICE (2024) recommendations and a local ear swabbing protocol.

Data collection: The electronic patient records and GP unit database were reviewed to extract data relevant to patients' clinical history, comorbidities, diagnostic ear swab tests and results, treatment provided and length of this, and follow-ups. The data was then transferred to the study's data collection spreadsheet. Data added corresponded to the pre-defined criteria for the audit.

The data was collated on a Microsoft excel spreadsheet and every patient added to the data collection spreadsheet was assigned a random identification number, ensuring patient anonymity.

Data analysis: The data was analysed by calculating the mean, mode, median, range, standard deviation and percentages. The analysed data was presented with the use of descriptive statistics, i.e. using tables, charts and graphs.

Ferreira provides some reflections on the audit (the management of otitis externa), the challenges involved and what could have been done differently in Box 5.2.

Box 5.2: Reflection on clinical audit study

Conducting this audit on the management of otitis externa using retrospective data from clinical records (secondary data analysis) proved challenging in some respects. The reliance on secondary data proved particularly time-consuming, as clinical documentation would vary greatly between clinicians and was recorded predominantly in free text. Missing or unclear entries frequently resulted in patient exclusion, reducing the overall dataset and resulted in increased labour/time spent. Future clinical audits could benefit from the analysis of more structured or closed-field documentation (e.g., prefilled templates, with yes/no options), which would streamline data extraction and enhance overall reliability. From my experience, I also noted that examining three different parameters of otitis management (i.e., antibiotic use, ear swabs and follow-up) also proved ambitious and increased complexity of the audit. At times, one parameter was well-documented while another was not, suggesting that focusing on one or two clearly defined variables might yield more robust conclusions (being very selective and focused in the study). Another key learning point was the need to recognise and account for confounding variables in this type of data analysis, such as ENT clinician experience or seniority, which may have led to variation in practice and influence outcomes. In hindsight, I could have allocated more time for data collection, which could be easier to do by a dedicated team rather than an individual. The use of a pre-configured data collection spreadsheet with closed fields (excel software, designed with drop down options) was a particularly effective tool for my audit, simplifying the process and allowing for rapid statistical analysis, and I would recommend future students to use this type of tool when doing this type of retrospective audit.

Points to consider:

- Make sure you have identified what information you are looking for before you start. In the example above, the first standard that the audit was looking to compare was 'cleaning the external ear canal from debris with micro suction and providing a 7- to 14-day course of topical antibiotics ear drops with or without topical steroids'. Therefore, data which was being identified from the patient records would have included:
  - Was the external ear canal cleared of debris with micro suction? (Yes/No or Missing)
  - Was a 7- to 14-day course of topical ear antibiotics prescribed? (Yes/No or Missing)
  - Was a 7- to-14-day course of topical steroids prescribed? (Yes/No or Missing)
- At the same time, you need to be precise about what data you need and ensure that you only access data for which you have permission to do so (via your ethical permission). This might seem a trivial point but there can be professional implications if you do not adhere to the procedures for extracting data. Therefore, careful planning of the data you need will prevent you from realising at a later date that you have missed some vital information during data collection.
- You will need to consider how you will capture and log the information you retrieve. Although you could use paper and pen to do this, it makes more sense to do this electronically both for safe storage of data and well as ease of use. Something as simple as a spreadsheet is all you need to start this process. You need to think about what information is needed and devise your criteria accordingly, then devise the columns in the spreadsheet to fit this information. Consider also how you will log missing data and whether there is an alternative way you can locate such information – although for small-scale projects this is unlikely. Figure 5.1 shows the data sheet used to capture the data extracted from the EPR records in the example above.
- Ensure strict adherence to the privacy and data protection principles that apply to your project, especially if doing an audit or service evaluation, where there is an expectation that you will be accessing patient data. If undertaking a small-scale research project, this will not necessarily apply, although there is a growing trend for healthcare facilities to ask for generic consent from patients and clients that their data can be used for research. However, it is important not to assume that this agreement is in place.

Sample number	Age (years)	Sex (M/F)	Ear swab taken? (Y/N)	Risk factors for NOE: 1) Age > 80 2) Disbetes 3) Immunocompromise	Ear swab indicated? 1) NOE risk factor 2) Recurrent or parsisant OE	Microbiology growth of ear swab sample	Oral antibiotics prescribed? (Y/N)	Oral antibiotics indicated?(Y/N) 1) severe OE 2) immunacompromised	Patient had follow-up appointment or re-attended? (Y/N)	Time of f/u from initial review (days)	Follow-up or re-attendance indicated?(Y/N) 1) severe OE 2) immunacompromised 3) unresolving symptoms or persistent symptoms - NICE (2024)
1											
2											
3											
4											
5											
6											
7											
8											
9											
10											
11											
12											
13											
14											
15											
16											
17											
18											
19											
20											
21											
22											
23											
24											
25											

Figure 5.1 Example data sheet.

Data collected via surveys and interviews

If you are undertaking a project using a survey and/or interviews, you will need to consider how you will *recruit* participants. How you go about this will be part of your ethical and other approvals, which we discuss in Chapter 4. You need to ensure that how you approach potential participants is as unobtrusive as possible and that no one feels coerced to take part. You also need to make your project as accessible as possible to potential participants. The point here is that you are *inviting* people to take part – they are not obligated to do so. There is also no obligation on the part of your colleagues to promote the study for you. This might mean your project going under the radar unless you can identify strategies that keep it in the forefront of people's minds.

Box 5.3: Recruitment of participants

Recruitment involves approaching potential participants directly (in person or by phone) or by inviting them to respond to a request for volunteers using posters, email, posts, flyers or leaflets (see Figure 5.2, an example from Birch 2024). Until recently, the most common way to advertise a study was via a poster or by word of mouth. Of course, now there are many opportunities to promote your study using social media and these are discussed by Wright et al. (2024). This can be via generic platforms such as X (formerly Twitter) or LinkedIn, or via specific interest groups. The advantages and disadvantages of using social media as a recruitment tool are explored by Oudat and Bakas (2023) and Jones et al. (2024). When you apply for ethical approval, your approach to potential participants will be scrutinised for any potential for undue influence or pressure to take part.

Once people have responded to an initial advertisement or promotion about the proposed study, the rest of the study recruitment will follow. In the posters or other means of advertisement, it's a good idea to include an electronic link such as a QR code that directs volunteers to the next steps, such as contact with the researcher to arrange an interview or to an online survey. All potential volunteers need to be fully informed and provide consent if they decide to participate, as discussed in Chapter 4.

Recruitment to a project can be challenging (Klompstra et al. 2025). This is in part due to guidelines and policies that govern your invitation to participate – for example, many institutions do not allow potential participants to be emailed directly. In addition, potential recruits need to be persuaded that it would be a good use of their time. Many initiatives have been undertaken in an attempt to improve recruitment (Kennedy et al. 2025; Milinic et al. 2025). Some have focused on achieving a representative sample by opening participation to groups not historically invited to take part in research, as discussed in Chapter 3. Such strategies, however, are likely to be beyond the scope and remit of someone doing a small-scale empirical project for whom recruiting enough participants will be challenging enough. These challenges can be described in your limitations section when writing up your project (see Chapter 7). Furthermore, if you are doing a small-scale empirical study, whether qualitative, quantitative or mixed methods, your sample size is likely to be limited by the scope of your project. However, you can still consider ways in which you can recruit a diverse sample rather than focusing on a group of people who are likely to tell you the same thing, again as we discussed in Chapter 3.

Once you have established your method of recruitment, think of how you can enhance this and how you can promote your study as widely as possible. Such strategies include:

- maintaining a presence in the area in which you are recruiting, assuming you have permission to be there;
- keeping in regular contact with anyone who is assisting your recruitment;
- asking others to re-circulate any social media advertisement of your project;
- keeping in touch with potential participants who have expressed an interest in your study.

If you are struggling to recruit participants, discuss this with your supervisor to identify if there are any strategies you can adopt to facilitate further interest in your project. There is a fine line between encouraging participants to take part and coercion – which is, of course, not permissible.

Data collected from surveys

'Survey' is the umbrella term used for gathering written or verbal information about people or situations for the purpose of analysing and interpreting data. The belief is that the best way to find out what's

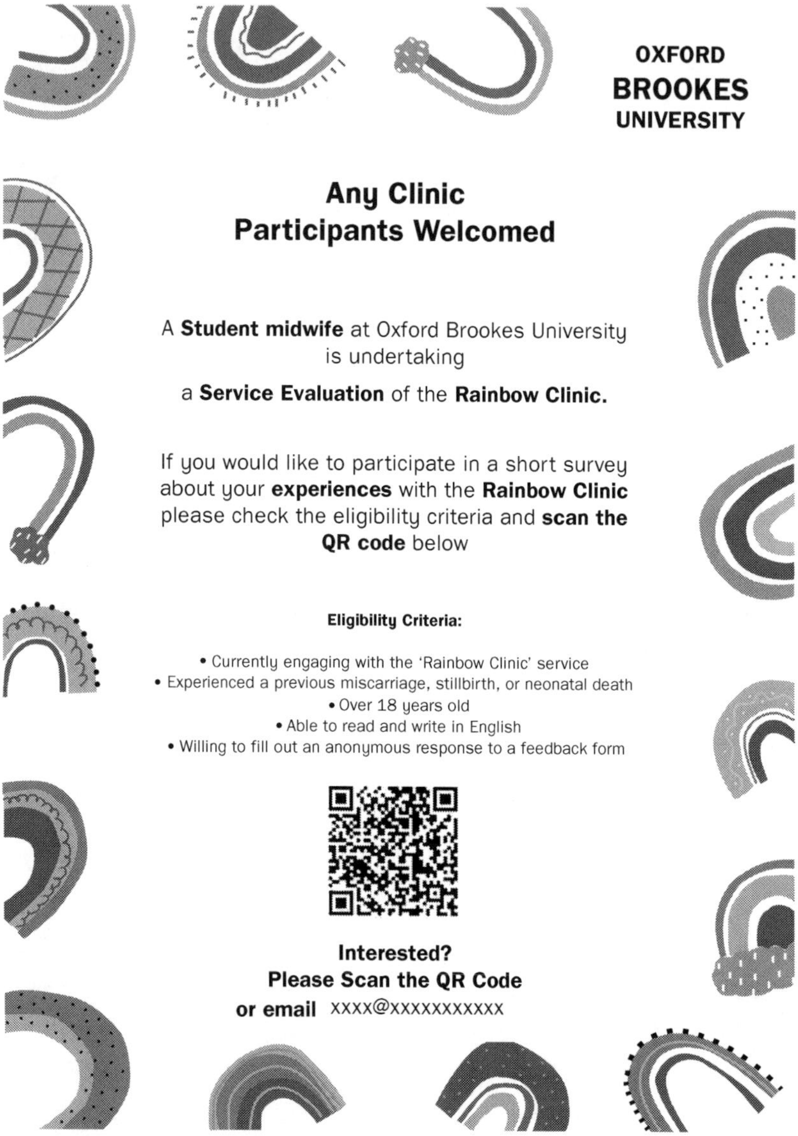

Figure 5.2 Example recruitment poster.

going on is to ask the people involved – this is the thinking behind most surveys. For large-scale projects, hundreds or even thousands of people can be involved, but this won't be the case for your audit, service evaluation or small-scale research project. Sometimes, respondents are asked to respond to a set of pre-determined questions. At other times, the researcher records information about the thing they are surveying, such as a traffic survey or a time-and-motion study. Generally, the information gathered is used to describe, identify patterns or trends, or make sense of a situation. This information will often be in the form of numbers. For example, your respondents might be asked to choose a number on a scale of, say, 1–5 to rate an experience or outcome – although increasingly qualitative data will form part of survey results. Strictly speaking, the first data collection method we described, using existing patient records, is also a type of survey.

A **questionnaire** is a type of survey that consists of a set of questions that are designed to collect specific information from your participants. Most often it will be a self-completed questionnaire, either a paper copy sent by post or, more common nowadays, an electronic or online version. The terms 'survey' and 'questionnaire' are often used interchangeably, although typically a questionnaire is a list of questions, whereas a survey is the process of using those questions to find something out. For example, you might want to conduct a survey to understand how satisfied patients are with their care, using a service evaluation or small-scale research project. In this case, you would use a questionnaire to collect the information and gather opinions that you can then draw together to answer your research question. There are limitations to using questionnaires which we discuss below, such as getting the design right and obtaining a large enough sample. For this reason, they may not be able to provide sufficient information to answer your question by themselves. They are often used together with other data collection methods (see the section on mixed methods below). For a comprehensive treatment of questionnaire development and research, we recommend the key text by Patten (2016) entitled *Questionnaire Research: A Practical Guide.*

There are multiple benefits of using questionnaires. Perhaps the most significant is that a questionnaire makes it possible to collect information from lots of participants quickly, with a reasonable amount of effort and at a low cost, particularly if distributed online. As all participants answer the same questions, this helps keep the results fair and consistent and reduces bias. Also, because the participants often complete questionnaires privately in their own time and space, they can do so when it is convenient for them and they are not rushed or distracted. They may also feel more comfortable about being honest in their responses, especially when asked about personal topics like mental health or habits such as smoking, diet or exercise. The survey may be designed to capture data at a single point in time (cross-sectional) or over multiple time points (longitudinal). That is, the questionnaire can be used more than once to see how things change over time, such as before and after a treatment or health programme, or in relation to service delivery.

As noted above though, questionnaires also have limitations, one of which is the possibility of a poor response rate. As one cannot require participants to respond, and many do not, most researchers must make do with only a small number of completed questionnaires. Although you won't know exactly who has responded, it is likely to be participants with similar characteristics. In this case, the data is unlikely to be representative of the target population. For example, if 30 per cent of the sample respond, we will never know how the other 70 per cent would have responded. If the questionnaire takes the form of an online survey, identifying the response rate won't be possible.

Furthermore, in today's world it seems we are constantly being asked to fill out marketing questionnaires and provide customer feedback – whether that's after buying something online, visiting a website or using an app. Because of this, many people become tired and annoyed by such requests. The frequent use of surveys to gather data has led many people to become increasingly reluctant to respond. This is called 'survey fatigue', whereby people either ignore any request to complete a questionnaire or rush through it, or even provide random answers just to finish quickly. Whilst this is of course entirely at the respondent's discretion, the key to the success of a questionnaire survey is to obtain a representative response rather than a skewed response based on a particular subset of people, for example patients who have had a negative experience and are keen to report this. This is why getting a representative sample of people to respond to a questionnaire is so important. A non-representative sample will be to the detriment of the study findings.

In questionnaire surveys, accurate and thoughtful answers are vital. It is possible that respondents misunderstood some of the questions, especially if the wording was complicated or used jargon or unfamiliar terms. This can lead to mistakes, incorrect or unclear answers, or even skipping questions altogether. And if the questionnaire is considered too long or perceived to be boring, there is a high likelihood the potential participant will simply discard it. This will result in no or poor-quality data and you won't have the opportunity to go back and ask the participant directly or be able to rephrase the question for them or ask any follow-up questions. So, questionnaire design is key, as we discuss below.

Identifying the right people to participate in your survey is vital. One means of doing so is to invite people to respond to an invitation or advertisement posted/hosted on a public or general media site. Remember that all your survey participants will by necessity be volunteers. They will need to be motivated to respond to your survey and be willing to take the time and effort required. A regular criticism of small-scale surveys is that respondents tend to be 'the usual suspects'. Put thought into targeting those who are most likely to be interested or affected by the topic you are investigating. In the example below (see Box 5.4), Lascelles (2024) first distributed her survey to contacts who were in a position to distribute it more widely to the people most likely to be interested and motivated to respond. Another tactic is to make your survey available to a specific population or populations only (if your study protocol allows; see Chapter 4).

Self-reported questionnaires also require the respondents to be able to read and write, so people with low literacy or language barriers may be excluded. Being able to ask survey questions in person and record the answers will overcome some of these issues, but this is a resource-intensive procedure (and goes against some of the advantages of self-completion).

The above points make clear that questionnaire design and construction is a complex undertaking. However, this is a problem you are unlikely to face if doing an audit. If you are undertaking a small-scale research project, it is easier and often far better to use an existing validated questionnaire, as it will have already been tested for reliability and validity and you will be able to compare your project with others that have used the same tool. If the questionnaire does not fit the cultural, contextual or language needs of the research, you can adapt it as necessary – remember to seek permission to do so from the original author of the questionnaire. Create a new one from scratch only as a last resort.

Once you have developed or adapted your questionnaire and consider it is ready to use, it will first need to be administered to a small group of people from your target population, ideally as part of your patient and public involvement and engagement (PPIE; see Chapter 3). This applies to the use of all questionnaires, regardless of whether you have developed it yourself. If that is not possible, you might ask a trusted friend, colleague or family member to do this for you. This step is called pilot testing, and it helps you check your questionnaire is fit for your purpose. The development of a questionnaire for research purposes can take years of work, and various methods and rounds of statistical testing will be required to demonstrate the final version is both valid (it measures what it is supposed to measure) and reliable (it provides consistent results over time). You will not have the means or time to do this for your small project, although pilot testing will be necessary. The feedback you get at this point will be valuable, indicating if any changes are necessary before you distribute your survey for real. Ask your testers to go through the questionnaire and point out anything they find confusing or unclear. If they spot any problems, or you notice them giving unusual or unexpected answers, take the time to revise and improve your questions or response options. Note if the answers they provide are useful for your project, and if not, replace or reformat those questions so that the answers they provide are relevant.

In summary, piloting will confirm your questionnaire is fit for purpose – that is, your testers are able to understand what they are being asked to do and can complete all the questions asked of them without issue. Consequently, it is more likely that your study participants will respond as you wish them to, thus leading to a better set of results.

Survey using an existing questionnaire

Our first example is of data collected using existing questionnaires. This is the most straightforward of questionnaire projects as you will be using an existing tool and do not need to worry about developing or adapting it yourself.

Lascelles (2024) undertook a mixed-methods research study within which pre-existing questionnaires were used to assess the needs of adult carers of adults at risk of suicide. The aim was to enhance understanding of the needs of this group of carers so that support for them could be delivered more effectively. This survey involved the use of five pre-existing and widely used questionnaires for measuring quality of life. As they had already been tested for reliability and validity, they were considered reliable tools for collecting this type of data from participants. Given that the sample in this research consisted of adult carers of adults at risk of suicide, pre-existing questionnaires could be used to measure quality of life in this population. There was no need to develop an additional tool, thus reducing the workload of the researcher substantially.

Ethical approval focused on the potential for harm to participants from completing the questionnaire. The participants were already in a difficult situation owing to their caring responsibilities, and it was important not to add to this burden. Interestingly, Lascelles included an extra, short questionnaire which addressed the burden of taking part in the study. This data was collected in order to evaluate the true risk of distress to participants in the study. Responses indicated that whilst participation was an emotional experience for many, this did not add to the overall burden of care and in fact many participants found the experience to be somewhat therapeutic (Lascelles 2024). This study provided additional evidence that questionnaires can be used to address complex and sensitive topics and do not necessarily add to distress – they might in fact help alleviate it. Lascelles' study is useful reading for anyone looking for evidence of potential harm to research participants and might be seen as rationale for the inclusion of a potentially vulnerable group in research, as we discussed in Chapter 4. The information obtained from participants who completed the existing questionnaire survey was supplemented with the use of interviews. Here we report only the method for doing the questionnaire survey.

Box 5.4: Example of a project in which data was collected via existing questionnaires

Title: Using Existing Questionnaires to Examine the Perceived Stigma and Quality of Life of Adult Carers Supporting Adults at Risk of Suicide.

Development of the survey: The questionnaire was developed from existing instruments: the Adult Carer Quality of Life scale (AC-QoL) (Elwick et al. 2010) and the Stigma of Suicide Attempt (STOSA) scale (Scocco et al. 2012). Additional closed and open questions specific to the research question and demographic questions were included. The main survey therefore consisted of questions regarding the carers' quality of life while caring for someone at risk of suicide. In addition, questions were asked about the carers' experience of completing the questionnaire, as it was about a distressing topic. These included pre- and post-survey mood ratings and additional open response questions.

Distribution of the survey: The researcher distributed the survey via their own and their employing NHS Trust's Twitter and Facebook accounts. In addition, local carer organisations and local and national professional contacts were approached and asked to distribute the online survey link to relevant individuals and groups via social media or by email. Four moderated Facebook carer and mental health nursing groups also agreed to advertise the survey on their sites. The invitation to participate was attached to an image and brief advertisement text outlining the purpose of the research and inviting eligible individuals to take part. When respondents clicked on the survey link, they were directed to the participant information followed by mandatory response informed consent questions. Eligibility questions followed consent and again these involved mandatory responses. If a response indicated non-eligibility, the respondent was taken via skipped logic to a section of the survey which confirmed the reason they were not eligible and provided information about relevant support agencies. The questionnaires took approximately 20–25 minutes to complete.

Completion rate: In no-restriction, self-selected surveys such as this, it is not possible to calculate a response rate because the number of people who had access to the survey cannot be known (Toepoel 2016). A completion rate is determined by subtracting the number of people who completed a survey from the number who started but did not complete it. In this study, the survey link was clicked for viewing 390 times. In total, 189 responses were commenced and this figure was taken to be the initial sample size. Eighteen participants were ineligible for the study. Seventy responses were excluded for being incomplete (i.e. respondents did not complete all the survey questions or any of the demographic questions, which was required for the analysis). The final survey sample was 101 respondents, or 53 per cent of the 189 individuals who commenced the survey.

Points to consider:

- The use of pre-existing questionnaires is ideal for small-scale research projects but less likely to be so for an audit or service evaluation where the survey needs to be designed specifically for the service in question. The benefit of using pre-existing questionnaires (sometimes rather confusingly known as 'survey scales') is that the questions have already been tested for validity and reliability; that is, we know that the questionnaire will be answered in a similar manner by different participants and that the questions asked will generate the data sought by the needs of the project. There are accessible and reliable questionnaires for various common outcomes that you may have chosen to measure: 'quality of life', 'patient satisfaction', 'levels of anxiety' or 'students' learning outcomes', such as the Study Process Questionnaire (SPQ). You can identify relevant questionnaires by undertaking a database search or even the judicious use of artificial intelligence.
- Whilst using a pre-existing (validated) questionnaire is ideal, of course one might not be relevant to your project. Where a pre-existing questionnaire is not suitable, it might be possible to modify one.

Discuss with your supervisor ahead of doing so, since any modifications will usually need to be agreed with the author of the questionnaire as these might lead to changes in how the questionnaire is received, and hence lessen the validity of the data collected and therefore the results.

Survey using an adapted questionnaire

Our next example involves collecting data using an adapted but pre-existing questionnaire. In this service evaluation, Guillermo-Scott (2025) was interested in the provision of person-centred care within a rehabilitation service. This student identified an existing validated tool – the Person-centred Care Assessment Tool (P-CAT), available at: https://www.dementiaresearch.org.au/resources/person-centred-care-assessment-tool-p-cat/

Guillermo-Scott examined the tool carefully to determine whether it was appropriate for their project. The original P-CAT aimed to measure the experience of providing person-centred care from the perspective of care home staff and has been used in many research projects internationally. Guillermo-Scott's service evaluation planned to look at the delivery of person-centred care from the perspective of a different group – that of carers in a rehabilitation service rather than a care home. The questionnaire was relevant but needed to be adapted to incorporate the perspectives of rehabilitation staff. The original questionnaire consisted of 13 statements about care: Guillermo-Scott's suggested adaptation involved including the word 'rehabilitation' as well as 'care' and because the original instrument was intended for care homes, that the word 'residents' should also be removed.

Points to consider:

- When you adapt an existing validated questionnaire for your own purposes, you need to seek permission from the original author of the tool.
- Once permissions have been obtained, acknowledge that you are altering a tool that has previously been tested for validity and reliability and any alterations you make might change the way the tool is responded to.
- Ideally, any adaptations ought to be tested in a pilot study. This is because you are changing a tool that has been developed to work in a certain way.

- Include a section on the effect that the adaptation might have had on your data collection and test this out if possible; if you do not have the resources to test the revised version, you cannot be sure of its validity and reliability and hence the usefulness of the data obtained.

Guillermo-Scott (2025) provided the following reflections on the data collection for their study in Box 5.5.

Box 5.5: Reflection on adapting questionnaires for data collection

If I was planning this study again, I would include a qualitative component, such as open-ended questions or short interviews, to complement the quantitative data gathered through the proposed adaptation of the validated Likert scale questionnaire (P-CAT). Whilst the quantitative data would provide measurable insights and facilitated statistical analysis, it limited the depth of understanding regarding the service evaluation participants' perspectives and experiences. Incorporating qualitative methods could have offered richer context and explanations for certain patterns in the quantitative findings.

One key pitfall to look out for when using adapted instruments is ensuring that the adaptation process does not compromise the validity or reliability of the original tool. It is also essential to pilot test the adapted questionnaire with a small group to confirm clarity, cultural relevance, and consistency of responses, which needs to be planned. Another challenge is ensuring an adequate response rate. In my case, this was improved through reminders and clear communication of the study's purpose.

For future students, I would recommend careful planning of data collection timelines, early ethics approval, permissions and pre-testing of instruments. Combining both quantitative and qualitative approaches can provide a more comprehensive understanding of the research topic and strengthen the overall quality of the findings.

Survey using a self-developed questionnaire

If there is no appropriate existing questionnaire, the next possibility is to construct your own. If your data collection is likely to be relatively straightforward, such as for an audit or service evaluation, this can be achieved within a reasonably short time frame. Where the data you need is more complex, the design of a questionnaire can become a project in its own right – and hence might be beyond the scope of your current project. You will need to spend time and effort in 'getting it right'. In this section, we will outline some of the general considerations for developing your own questionnaire. Of course, if you want to do this you should consult a reputable text to guide you (e.g. Jones and Rattray 2015) and take advice, as always, from your project supervisor or another expert.

Developing your own questionnaire

The questions asked should always be designed with your research question in mind, but the types of questions and how they are worded is also significant. Closed questions involve respondents choosing their answer based on a limited number of predefined responses, such as a binary response ('yes/no') or multiple-choice options. For example, 'Have you been diagnosed with hypertension (high blood pressure)?' – no / yes / don't know.

You need to provide sufficient options, as otherwise the question may be ignored completely, or an answer selected that only partly meets a respondent's desired response. For example, multiple-choice options for 'how did you travel here today?' might be 'car', 'walk', 'bus' or 'train', but there is no option for 'electric scooter' or 'tram'. Providing an 'other' option with space to jot down (or type) their preferred response would be useful here. Also, you could allow respondents to select more than one option, in case they use more than one method of transport. Alternatively, you may want to limit them to one answer, and so would need to make it clear in the question that what you are asking for is their main mode of transport only.

Making sure your questions are acceptable in terms of their meanings and inclusivity is also important. For example, it is no longer considered acceptable to ask participants to choose between male or female when defining their gender. Instead, you might ask: 'Which of the following best describes your gender? Female, Male, Prefer to self-describe: __________ or Prefer not to say'. The literacy and language barriers we raised earlier are another factor; if you know your intended participants speak and read another language, then you need to provide them with a translated version of your English language questionnaire.

Open-ended questions such as 'What would you say are the best things about this centre?' invite participants to respond in their own words and the inclusion of free-text boxes for their answer will accommodate this. This captures qualitative data which can be analysed appropriately alongside the more common quantitative responses. Free-text boxes can also be provided after a closed question, in order to allow for an explanation. For example, 'if you answered no – please explain your response in the box below'.

Lastly, other questions often used in questionnaires ask respondents to rate their experiences or opinions of things according to a scale, such as a Likert scale. A typical example of this is where a respondent is asked their opinion of a statement on a scale of 1–5, where 1 represents 'strongly agree' and 5 represents 'strongly disagree'. Another question might ask, 'Overall, how would you rate your experience today?', where the means of response is to tick one of a series of boxes provided: 1 = 'Excellent', 2 = 'Good', 3 = 'Fair', 4 = 'Poor', and 5 = 'Very Poor'. Finally, you might decide to use visual aids to complete this sort of scale, for example using emoticons representing the feelings from 'happy' through 'neutral' to 'unhappy':

The wording of questions should be clear, concise and jargon-free. You want your participants to easily understand the questions and not be confused by any ambiguous wording. You should ask yourself if the questions you are asking are interesting and relevant to your likely participants. Expression will be key, so maintain a neutral tone – avoid any leading questions and steer clear of making your personal opinions apparent. It is important that respondents feel able to answer questions truthfully and not provide answers they deem to be 'correct' or what they believe the investigator (i.e. you) wants. Occasionally, people may choose not to answer truthfully or have a strong agenda of their own that affects their answers.

Think carefully about the order of questions, as it is best to build up from easier, more general and accessible questions to those that need much more thought and engagement. More sensitive topics might be better placed towards the end of the questionnaire. Remember that you will not have long to keep the attention of your participants, so while the questionnaire needs to be long enough to accommodate your need to acquire data, it should also be as brief as possible to maintain the respondents' interest.

The questionnaire's design can also have a positive effect on the completeness of data capture, for example by only allowing one box to be selected or forcing respondents to supply at least one answer to all questions before they can exit the survey (if in electronic format). A word of warning though: these rules can be incredibly annoying if applied vigorously, and you may lose the goodwill (and participation) of your respondents if you overstep this. Including a statement thanking participants for their time goes without saying.

The example we use for data collected using a self-developed questionnaire is from a service evaluation adapted from the work of Birch (2024). The aim of this service evaluation was to evaluate the experience of older adult users of a community day centre run by a charitable organisation. An anonymous questionnaire was designed to provide feedback from the users about their experiences at the centre in order to improve it. This is a good example of the sort of situation where it might be appropriate to develop a bespoke questionnaire. The student needed to ask simple questions of the users of the day centre which would not have been possible using a pre-existing questionnaire.

Box 5.6: Example of a project in which data was collected by self-developed questionnaire

Title: A Service Evaluation of the Twice Weekly Drop-in Sessions for Older Adults at a Community Centre.

Aim: This study investigated the experiences of the users of a community day centre for older adults, open on two days a week, run by a charitable organisation. The focus of the study was to identify who was accessing the sessions at the centre and whether these were meeting the needs of the service users.

Method: A survey design using a self-developed questionnaire.

Data collection: The adults accessing any of the drop-in sessions were invited to participate in the survey. Posters and leaflets advertising the survey were displayed in the centre's reception area and in the main activity room. The questionnaire was available to them electronically via a link (QR code) in the posters and leaflets, intended to be accessed by mobile phone. The link directed users to the participant information page followed by a consent form page. Respondents were unable to proceed with the questionnaire until consent was provided.

Paper versions of the questionnaire were also provided by staff to any service users who volunteered to complete the survey and preferred this method or could not access the electronic version. The paper version also included participant information and an anonymous consent box. All responses were confirmed as anonymous and no identifying data collected. The survey was open for six weeks.

The questions ranged from those asking for demographic information (e.g. age, sex, ethnicity) to open questions with free-text boxes for participants' feedback about their opinions of the sessions.

Data analysis: *Responses to the survey questions were analysed by descriptive statistics and thematic analysis as appropriate.*

An example of the type of short questionnaire that could be developed for this purpose is shown in Figure 5.3.

Community Centre questionnaire

Q1: What is your age?

____

Q2: What is your ethnicity?
Please choose one option from the following that best describes your ethnic group or background

- ○ White
- ○ Black / African / Caribbean / Black British
- ○ Mixed / Multiple ethnic groups
- ○ Asian / Asian British
- ○ Other ethnic group, please describe____________

Q3: What is your sex?

- ○ Male
- ○ Female
- ○ Non-binary / third gender
- ○ Prefer not to say

Q4: For how long have you been coming to the bi-weekly sessions at the centre?
Please choose one of the following options

- ○ This is my first time
- ○ Less than 6 months
- ○ Between 6 months and 1 year
- ○ Over a year

Figure 5.3 Example community centre questionnaire.

Q5: On average, how often do you go to the drop-in sessions at the centre? Please choose one of the following options

◯ 1 or 2 times a week

◯ 1 or 2 times each month

◯ Up to 6 times a year

◯ This is my first visit

Q6: Overall, on a scale of 1 to 5, how satisfied are you with the sessions at the centre? Please select one of the following

_____ Extremely dissatisfied
_____ Somewhat dissatisfied
_____ Neither satisfied nor dissatisfied
_____ Somewhat satisfied
_____ Extremely satisfied

Q7: Please tell us, what do you like about sessions at the centre?

Q8: Please tell us, is there anything that would improve your experience with these sessions at the centre?

Figure 5.3 *(Continued)*

Q9: Is there any further feedback you would like to give that you feel relevant?

Thank you for your time spent taking this survey

Your response has been recorded

Figure 5.3 (*Continued*)

Points to consider:

- Remembering the issues of poor completion and low response rates, it was important to make sure this questionnaire was reasonably short, clear and meaningful, so that the participants were more likely to take the questions seriously and respond in full. The questionnaire contained just 14 questions, some of which were very straightforward ('How old are you?'), and therefore did not take too long to complete. In this study, most people who started the questionnaire completed it, indicating its design and length were unproblematic for most.

- In this example the questionnaire was provided both as paper copies as well as electronically to demonstrate inclusive practice and to avoid digital exclusion. This raises another issue – that of finance. Before you start your project, you will need to consider the financial cost of printing and copying documents and posters; providing multiple paper copies of questionnaires might well be beyond your budget.

Questionnaires in experimental designs

So far, we have not paid much attention to study designs which are considered experimental in nature, where your project aims to test an idea or hypothesis. As we mentioned in Chapter 1, these types of projects will generally be outside the scope of this book's intended readership because they require much greater resources (such as equipment, medications, time, planning, personnel, and so on), although you may wish to conduct a type of small-scale experimental study. Interestingly, an audit (and to a lesser extent service evaluation) includes a hypothesis that is being tested, namely that the thing being measured will meet a particular standard.

An example of a larger-scale experimental study is where participants are randomised into one of two groups: a group that receives a particular intervention and a group that does not – that is, a randomised controlled trial (RCT). The observed outcomes for the two groups can be compared to determine whether the intervention was successful. The data is usually collected by means of a survey of the outcomes, which of course can be a self-completed questionnaire. The outcomes might also be measurements, such as weight loss or degree classification, and this data could be recorded and entered into the questionnaire by the researcher instead. Whilst an RCT is likely to be beyond the scope of anyone undertaking a small-scale research project, there are modified versions of this approach that might be used. The following is a pre- and post-test design.

Box 5.7: Meaning of observational study
From what we have just described, this is why some study designs are called 'observational' – note the meaning of observation here is very different to qualitative 'participant observation'.

The example we give here, using data collected by a questionnaire to inform an experimental project design, is based on a published paper by Bothra et al. (2025). This educational project used a pre-/post-test experimental design to evaluate the effectiveness of an intervention, a one-day thesis workshop, attended by postgraduate student participants in India. The effectiveness of the intervention was assessed by pre- and post-test questionnaires. Researchers developed the questionnaire themselves as it needed to be specific to evaluate the thesis writing workshop. It was piloted within the faculty among staff and students though there is no evidence of further testing to demonstrate validity and reliability. Note that there was no control group (students not receiving the intervention), making this a quasi-experiment – an adaptation of a RCT.

Points to consider:

- The questionnaire to test the knowledge and confidence developed by participants after a focused thesis writing workshop was developed specifically for the project.
- It is unclear to what extent the questionnaire was piloted but we are told that it was developed using the input of colleagues and students in faculty.
- Before and after measures do not necessarily measure the effectiveness of the intervention – there could be differences after the intervention that are not a result of the intervention itself.
- We cannot ascertain causality from a before and after experimental design, but such designs give us some understanding of the usefulness of an intervention.

Interviews for data collection

Data collection via a survey will likely focus on numerical, quantitative data. When the data that can be collected using a questionnaire is not sufficiently in-depth or detailed, qualitative data can be gathered directly from participants by means of an interview. Of course, a survey can involve the collection of information directly from participants too – a market researcher, for example, might phone you to ask if you would mind answering some questions – but an interview has the possibility of producing richer and more detailed data than this. Some sources describe all interviews as 'in-depth' to differentiate them from other forms of direct data collection.

Interviews are probably the most well-known method for collecting qualitative data. The verbal responses given to questions asked in an interview will be in the form of narratives, descriptions and words. Interviews are usually conducted either face-to-face, by phone or online, most often on a one-to-one basis. Interviews with a group of people conducted and facilitated by an interviewer are referred to as focus groups. The interview is recorded and then transcribed for analysis. An interview generally involves the articulation of people's thoughts, feelings, opinions and experiences, and these might be shaped by the way the interview is conducted. This information can help to explore and shed light on the topic at hand in a more in-depth way than quantitative data. Refer back to Chapter 3 as a reminder of the purpose behind your chosen method of data collection.

Another advantage of interviews is that there is less likely to be any misinterpretation; any misunderstandings can be clarified by the interviewer, thus helping to ensure completeness of the data. Interviews also allow the researcher to reach a wider audience, such as people with a visual impairment or poor literacy. The benefits of taking part in interview research has also been documented, including the fact that participants recall feeling listened to (McCallum 2022). However, because of their in-depth nature and quality, interviews are time-consuming, each interview lasting between 40 and 90 minutes. And despite most people being familiar with the format, interviewing is a highly skilled activity. These aspects are sometimes overlooked at the study design stage. For a comprehensive look at interviewing and its techniques, we recommend the key text by Kvale (1996) entitled *InterViews: An Introduction to Qualitative Research Interviewing*.

Let us now take a closer look at both individual interviews and focus groups.

Individual interviews

Interviews can be anywhere on the continuum between structured and unstructured. How you choose to conduct and structure your interview will depend on the aim of your project and will have a strong bearing on the responses you obtain, and how you analyse your data. Highly structured interviews, which are essentially a list of questions to be answered, are more like a survey and usually fall outside the pure qualitative domain. The respondent does not have the opportunity to go into any depth or provide information other than what is directly asked of them. Less structured interviews are usually based on standard questions, which make up an interview schedule or guide, which are asked of all respondents, but there is also space for the interviewer to ask follow-up questions, to probe for answers and to seek clarification if necessary. Therefore, it is possible to obtain a better insight into an interviewee's thoughts, understandings and perceptions. You will come across sources that collectively refer to these as 'semi-structured' interviews and this method will be most appropriate for small-scale projects. An example of an interview guide is given in Box 5.8 (adapted from Pugh 2023).

Box 5.8: Example interview guide/schedule

Interview guide: Providing Early Years (0–5 Years) Care for Children of Asylum-seeking Families Project.

About the job

Can you tell me what providing care for children of these families involves for you on a daily basis? (Prompt: key responsibilities, balancing other caseloads, differences with other service users)

Reflecting back to the beginning

How did you feel when you first learnt you would be looking after asylum-seeking families? (Prompt: Why did you feel that way? Can you tell me more about ...)

Can you tell me about any aspects that were initially challenging or concerning?

How did you approach/solve them?

Do you still consider them to be challenging?

Can you tell me about any support available to you in this work? (Prompt: Is there anything that would have been of benefit?)

How gaining experience informs the approach to care

Can you tell me about any strategies you have developed over time to help provide this care? (Prompt: What led you to do this? Cultural differences?)

Personally, how have you found the experience of providing this type of care?

> **Looking forward**
>
> How do you feel about providing care to asylum-seeking families in the future? (Prompt: What has influenced this? What could improve this?)
>
> What advice would you give to a colleague who is new to providing care to asylum-seeking families?

Even greater depth can be achieved by conducting a non-standardised or fully unstructured interview, which enables the participant to really tell their story. This approach requires a huge amount of skill and methodological rigour on the part of the interviewer, for example as part of phenomenological inquiry. In this approach a question could be as general as 'Tell me about your experience of sepsis', followed by several prompts to invite the interviewee to elaborate; as you can see the questions in this sort of interview develop from what the participant describes as being relevant or meaningful. Such an approach is much more likely to be used as part of a more theoretically driven study and would require a solid philosophical underpinning to the study design. If you are considering using interviews as a method of data collection, ensure that the type of interview that you select – structured, semi-structured or unstructured – is in line with the aim of your project.

Interviews are clearly used to obtain rich and illuminating data that would not be achievable using a survey method. This can be greatly enhanced by how the interview is conducted. The late Steiner Kvale (1996) saw interviews as a kind of conversation where meaning is created between interviewer and interviewee. He described the interviewer as being like a miner, digging out valuable information, or a traveller, going on a journey with the interviewee. These images are useful to help you move away from thinking of an interview as just simply a question-and-answer session, but instead a collaborative conversation between two people.

You should avoid asking closed questions to which participants can give a one-word or very short answer. The questions ought to be phrased simply, so their meaning is clear, and only one question should be asked at a time. You should be cognisant of your own influence on the interview, so avoid leading questions and responding over-enthusiastically to an answer. As the interviewer, you will need to listen carefully and pay attention not only to the words but to tones and pauses, while ensuring your behaviour and body language are neutral.

The interview will need to be recorded, either through online meeting software on a computer, or using a recording device (e.g. a Dictaphone) placed somewhere unobtrusive – remember, you want the participant to forget they are being recorded so they speak openly and freely. The quality of the recording is important as you will need to produce a transcript of the recorded interview later, so if conducting a face-to-face interview, make sure the equipment you use is working properly and have a back-up plan should any technical problems arise. Also, the interview will need to be conducted somewhere where you will not be disturbed and that allows your interviewee privacy. Conducting an interview in the corner of a teaching room or at a patient's bedside, for example, would not be a good idea.

A very important aspect of interviewing is confidentiality and ensuring that the interviewee cannot be identified from the transcript. Although you will replace their name with a pseudonym in the transcript, you also need to ensure that they, or any other individuals for that matter, cannot be identified from any other details. For example, you would certainly need to attend to the following: '*I'm Canadian and my accent is pretty strong. When I went to my very first placement – on a urology ward at the local hospital – I was told by the Sister in charge* ...', since both the interviewee and others are likely identifiable. This will also show respect for your interviewee and significantly you will want the interview to be an accurate account of what they said. This point is worth bearing in mind when you come to the analysis stage, as you will want the data to speak for themselves, at least to a certain extent, and therefore you must not manipulate or edit the transcript (beyond editing out personal details).

You could also consider offering your interviewees the chance to check the interview transcript for themselves, which is called 'member-checking'; however, this will create additional governance and methodological issues. Instead, it is good practice to indicate to all participants where they will be able to see the findings from your study, such as as a short summary on a named public-facing website.

The example we use for data collected using interviews is of a small-scale research project undertaken as part of a doctorate in education by Maddison (2023), who conducted in-depth interviews with a small number of participants, exploring how the past experiences and clinical context of practice assessors in nursing impacted their judgement of student nurses' performance (see Box 5.9). An interview guide was created to provide some structure and order for the questions to be asked, although the interviewer remained flexible in the approach to this, enabling participants' accounts to come to the fore. It was important for the participants to tell their stories in their own words as this perspective was central to the study's aims.

Box 5.9: Example of a project in which data was collected via interview

Title: The Impact of Clinical Context on the Practice Assessor's Perception of the Student Nurse's Performance on Placement: An Exploratory Narrative Inquiry.

Background: Literature – which was from the perspective of students – suggested that assessment of student nurses could be subjective, influenced by social processes like the student's personality, conformity, and interaction style – or their ability to 'fit in' – rather than solely objective standards. Less attention was given to how the practice assessors' own experiences and context might influence judgements.

Aims: To establish how practice assessors' experiences, including their clinical background, the context and the clinical environment impact their perception and judgement of student nurses' performance in clinical placements.

Method: The study adopted a narrative inquiry approach, which is interested in the experience of people and their accounts of experiences in the context of social, cultural, and environmental factors. Participants were six registered nurses in the field of adult nursing, practising in a clinical setting that supports pre-registration student nurses.

Data collection: To capture authentic narratives and to avoid the interviewer influence, the study utilised 1:1 interviews with a conversational style. An interview guide ensured focus and flexible question adjustment based on participant responses.

Data analysis: Core story creation was used to structure and condense the narratives into coherent, shorter accounts.

Results: The assessors' clinical context and experience impact judgement, leading to tacit assessment criteria based on the fit between proficiencies and the clinical area. Students with context-specific dispositions assimilate and succeed more easily. Broader socio-political factors also influence assessor attitudes and judgements.

Points to consider:

- Although a skilful interviewer will be flexible in their questioning, it remains important for there to be a clear purpose for the interview. You should know what it is you are seeking to find out, even if your study is largely exploratory in nature. As we explained previously regarding survey methods, piloting the interview guide and seeking feedback on the questions you intend to ask is good practice. You can do this with anyone willing to help you, although it you should not use this data in the analysis if the practice interview was undertaken ahead of the formal permissions process.

- It can be surprisingly awkward to conduct an interview for data collection purposes, and you may feel rather self-conscious and anxious doing so, particularly the first few times. This is another reason to conduct a pilot or rehearsal with a trusted friend or colleague. Experienced interviewers are confident in allowing enough time for their interviewees to respond fully to questions, and that silences are perfectly okay (they can result in more detailed responses).
- As with all research methods, ethical considerations are vital; issues of consent and trust are especially important to ensure that interviewees feel safe to share their experiences openly and that their rights are protected (see Chapter 4). In the example above, the interviewer was also a senior member of staff within the institution, so consideration had to be given to the appropriateness of interviewing currently enrolled students. In view of this Maddison (2023) invited students from a different campus and from different universities to participate, hence negating the conflict of interest that might have arisen if they had invited students who were part of her remit.

Focus group interviews

As we indicated earlier, a focus group is a type of interview undertaken with a small group of people who meet the criteria for your study. A focus group is conducted when it is anticipated that the discussion generated by the group will add to the richness of the data. Participants will have something in common, such as all being nursing students, or looking after partners with diabetes, or attending a particular clinic, and so on. The focus group is where they come together to talk about their experiences in a guided discussion, also called a guided interview. Often it can be more relaxed and informal in tone than a one-on-one interview, as the group leads much of the conversation. Usually, there are between four and ten participants and your role as the facilitator or moderator is to guide the conversation by asking key, open-ended questions. The intention of focus groups is less about individual experiences and more about the group's discussion of the topic and their shared insights and meanings. The group setting helps some people to express their views more openly than when one-on-one. And being in the company of others who share things in common makes the process more inclusive and welcoming. For more about focus group methodology, we recommend the key text by Liamputtong (2011), entitled *Focus Group Methodology: Principles and Practice*.

The main challenge to running a focus group is to coordinate potential participants' availability, which is especially pertinent if you do not have the resources to reimburse participants' time. You could consider naturally arising groups among which you might be able to undertake your study, but you need to bear in mind that no one should feel compelled to take part.

Once you have decided to run a focus group, the next step is to come up with your questions. These should be open-ended questions that encourage group discussion and help you explore the topic in more detail. The aim is to get people talking, sharing their thoughts and experiences, while also helping you gather the information you need. There are similar considerations to be made as for individual interviews. Piloting questions with a colleague or friend to gain feedback before you run a focus group with your intended participants is vital. Issues of confidentiality are similarly important when transcribing data, but an extra step is to remind all participants about confidentiality at the beginning of the focus group encounter because they will also be privy to the details that their co-participants share with the group.

The focus group questions should be created to encourage the group to talk to each other rather than asking the moderator to explain things or for their opinion. The aim is to keep the discussion moving along and prompting when you feel the time is right or the discussion is flagging or becoming faded. You should ensure all participants have a chance to speak and try to avoid a single individual from dominating the group.

As a general rule, a focus group should run for approximately an hour and no longer than 90 minutes or else your respondents will become fatigued. You should also consider where and how to host the group – it could be online, or if it's in person you will need to identify a convenient, quiet location, ideally where there won't be any interruptions. Either way, your participants should be made to feel at ease and comfortable so that a good collaborative atmosphere is created.

Having a colleague present at a focus group could help you facilitate the group – for example, they could note down the body language and other non-verbal clues of participants. For smaller or student-led projects, this will likely not be the case. Although it is easier to make notes if the focus group is run online, the advantages of conducting an in-person event will probably outweigh this. How you decide to conduct your focus group will likely be based on practicalities.

Sometimes, focus groups are used as a first step before carrying out one-to-one interviews. This is because the group discussion can help pinpoint the main themes, ideas or issues that matter most to participants and what language they use to talk about their experiences. This information can then be used to design better, more focused interview questions for individual interviews. In this way, the focus group helps shape the direction of the research and ensures that later questions are relevant and meaningful.

The example we use for interview data collected using focus groups is from a small-scale research project undertaken by Okiki et al. (2023) (see Box 5.10). This was part of a wider project by Okiki and colleagues (2023), who explored recruitment to midwifery programmes in England. The focus group interviews explored the experiences of Black, Asian and Minority Ethnic midwifery students at three universities in the southeast of England, where cohorts were predominantly White. Five virtual focus groups were conducted, facilitated by the lead author, with fourteen participants in total.

Box 5.10: Example of a project in which data was collected via focus group interviews

Title: 'Only for the White': A Qualitative Exploration of the Lived Experiences of Black, Asian and Minority Ethnic Midwifery Students.

Background: An ethnically diverse workforce has been identified as a key component of safe, compassionate maternity care, and yet midwifery remains a predominantly White profession across the Global North. Understanding the experiences of Black, Asian and Minority Ethnic midwifery students is key to addressing this disparity.

Aim: To capture the university and placement experiences of Black, Asian and Minority Ethnic midwifery students in a culturally White environment.

Methods: A qualitative study undertaken with student midwives studying at three separate universities in the southeast of England. Data were gathered through focus groups, conducted as part of a wider project looking at recruitment to midwifery programmes in England. Five virtual focus groups and two semi-structured interviews were conducted and recorded with thirteen current student midwives and one recent graduate self-identifying as Black, Asian or Minority Ethnic. Focus group discussions lasted around 60 minutes and were guided by open and prompt questions. Participants were invited to consider how their ethnicity had affected their experiences as students in university and on placement.

All current and recently graduated students at participating universities were emailed an invitation to participate together with a participant information sheet. Prospective participants needed to self-identify as belonging to a Black, Asian or Minority Ethnic group. Interested participants contacted the first author and were given a range of focus group dates to attend and a written consent form to return. When only one participant could attend, an individual interview was conducted instead. Contributors could ask for particular comments not to be included in the transcript of their focus group, and one comment was deleted due to a participant request. No participants withdrew from the study. Responses in focus groups are reported as a response from the group; this further protects the anonymity of participants.

Findings: Although some participants reported positive experiences and felt well supported, an overarching narrative emerged of midwifery as an exclusive and White profession. Institutionalised Whiteness was experienced in university, on placement and within individual student cohorts. Four themes were identified: 'being an outsider', 'prejudice, discrimination and racism', 'nowhere to turn' and 'positive forces'.

Okiki provided some reflections on the focus group interviews, the challenges involved and what they might have done differently (see Box 5.11) (C. Okiki, personal communication, October 29, 2025).

Box 5.11: Reflection on focus group interviewing: experiences of Black, Asian and Minority Ethnic midwifery students at three universities in the southeast of England

Challenges

Balancing empathy with maintaining the focus of the interview. For some participants, the session served as a reflective space or even their first outlet for expression and interrupting them would have felt unkind.

Maintaining the right level of control to prevent stories from dominating. But at times discussions went off topic, and in some cases this enabled quieter participants to find entry points into the conversation. They often contributed more effectively as part of those evolving discussions than in direct response to prompt questions.

Building towards the key investigative question on discrimination, which we had strategically placed halfway through the session.

Encountering harmful experiences that required attention and determining how to remain within the ethical boundaries of the study while supporting participants and maintaining confidentiality, particularly in situations where participants were uncertain about the outcomes they desired from their disclosures.

Being careful to remind everyone of maintaining confidentiality outside the focus group, e.g. some participants worked in the same practice setting.

Managing the huge sense of perceived responsibility that accompanies any exploration or investigation.

Things I wish I had approached differently

Seeking both short-term and long-term psychological support, for myself, due to the nature of the study. Listening to the experiences repeatedly during transcription.

Managing the length of personal stories more effectively. Many participants who may have lacked prior opportunities for expression used the session as a reflective space, resulting in very long narratives.

Ensuring safety in virtual sessions, including verifying that participants had access to appropriate devices and stable internet connections. Transcribing recordings made with poor internet coverage was a nightmare.

Keeping a diary of my own experiences and reflections following each focus group session.

Okiki also provided some practical tips for anyone considering conducting a focus group (see Box 5.12).

Box 5.12: Practical tips for conducting a focus group

1. Begin with an icebreaker that includes a personal touch – it can be very effective. Why should they share with you? What is the point anyway?

2. Allow flexibility in timing and in the flow of questions.
3. Clearly communicate all expectations and next steps both at the beginning and at the end of each session, and how they can contact you in the future.
4. Should you disseminate the work, try to ensure your participants are amongst the first to know the outcome of their contributions.
5. Be open to participants recommending sessions to friends (late joiners); flexibility in the recruitment period can be beneficial.
6. At times, nobody will volunteer to speak first, or to speak at all. Allow the silence to exist. Prepare a wide range of prompting questions and be ready to 'proceed and revisit' questions if participants are not yet prepared to respond.

Points to consider:

- Your main consideration when planning a focus group study will be the practicalities of getting a group of people together for the interview: convening a group of people is much more difficult to manage than arranging an individual interview. This can be helped by the offer of a small incentive, but this is likely to be beyond your means for a small-scale project. Conducting an online meeting, as in the example above, tends to be easier to organise than in-person focus groups.
- It is recommended to have at least four participants so that no one feels 'put on the spot', and any perceived pressure to speak is shared. Conversely, too many voices can make it harder for everyone to join in; quieter voices or those with a minority opinion could feel stifled, thus limiting the quality of the discussion. In the example above, the focus groups had only two or three participants, so there was no issue regarding being able to contribute.
- The focus group moderator, who was Black, had been a midwifery student, something that the participants could identify with, helping them to feel at ease and promoting honest reflection and debate.
- That the data produced was credible was demonstrated by the gathering of perspectives from multiple universities and across cohorts, and the use of in-group member checking where the moderator summarised and paraphrased participants words back to them in order to ensure she understood them correctly.

In the above example, despite offering participants a choice in arrangements, on occasion only one participant attended and so an individual interview was conducted instead. Here, this was a good contingency plan, but it would not be appropriate if the purpose of data collection was to gather the points of view of a group of participants.

The moderator in this example had knowledge of some of the things discussed in the interviews, so it was imperative that she remained neutral and focused on the participants' perspectives of these. This can be done by the moderator setting aside their personal experiences and viewpoints, and by discussion and debriefing with project supervisors.

Combining different methods of data collection

As we stated at the start of this chapter, some projects may use more than one method of data collection. Projects where both numerical (quantitative) and non-numerical (qualitative) data are captured and analysed are generally described as using a mixed-methods approach, although a project that uses two qualitative methods – for example, individual interviews and focus groups – might also be considered mixed methods.

A common mixed-methods design is to use both a survey and interviews to address a research question. Proponents of this approach argue that using a combination of the two methods will provide a fuller picture than either one could on its own (Creswell and Creswell 2023). However, the task of combining the different datasets should not be underestimated, or the understanding needed of the types of research question that can be addressed using a mixed-methods protocol. A general guide is that quantitative data is used to answer 'what' questions, and qualitative data 'why' or 'how' questions. It is important when using mixed methods that the research question clearly seeks to understand both a situation ('what') and its meaning (the 'why/how') (Wasti et al. 2022). The underlying philosophy to the bringing together of the two types of questions is called pragmatism, and while going into this may be beyond the scope of the readership of this book, you should make yourself familiar with its main principles, as discussed in Chapter 1. There is also much criticism of the use of mixed-methods research that lacks methodological rigour. An example of a well-received published mixed-methods paper is that by Desborough et al. (2016), who investigated how Australian nursing care practices affect patient satisfaction. The 'what' question about the nursing service was addressed by a survey, while the 'why' question was explored by individual interviews with patients. A key text for mixed-methods research is that of Creswell (2022), entitled *A Concise Introduction to Mixed Methods Research*.

The example we use of data collected using two different methods is from a service evaluation undertaken to explore women service users' experiences and outcomes at a sexual health clinic (see Box 5.13). This project was adapted from the work of Widdows (2022).

Box 5.13: Example of a project using a mixed-methods approach

Title: A Mixed-Methods Service Evaluation of the Experiences and Outcomes for Women Users of a Sexual Health Clinic.

Background: After a first appointment at the clinic, the women were given information about contraception and offered intrauterine contraception – either a copper intrauterine device (IUD) or hormonal intrauterine system (IUS). Women who had received any intrauterine contraception between March 2020 and November 2021 were contacted by letter with a phone call follow-up and asked to complete a questionnaire about their experiences. Those who agreed to the survey and completed it were further invited to be interviewed.

Data collection: Survey outcome measures were satisfaction, side effects, pathway effectiveness, continuation and expulsion rates. Sixty-one women completed the questionnaire, and four women consented to an online interview.

Results: Six weeks after the contraception was fitted, there were four cases of expulsion, with a total of eight being reported by 6 months. The continuation rate was 86.6% (n = 41) at 6 weeks and 76.8% (n = 33) at 6 months. Overall satisfaction was high with 75.5% (n = 43) of the women reporting they were either 'extremely satisfied' or 'somewhat satisfied'. All participants required additional follow-up in a primary care setting. No cases of uterine perforation or pregnancy were reported.

A thematic analysis of the interview data was performed with two main themes emerging: 'pressurised decision-making' (related to the effectiveness and timing of information) and 'post contraception transition' (follow-up and experiences of coming to terms with intrauterine contraception). Findings emerging from both the interview data and questionnaire were synthesised.

Conclusion: This service evaluation found that the provision of intrauterine contraception at the clinic was effective with good continuation rates; however, recommendations are made for future improvement of the service including better contraception counselling and follow-up.

Points to consider:

- The findings of this service evaluation show that the service users of the clinic were either 'extremely satisfied' or 'somewhat satisfied' with their care (contraception service), something which could have been measured by a survey alone. However, the four interviewees provided more in-depth information about their experiences, outside of the specific questions asked, and so this data contributed to a more complete understanding of service user experience. Overall, it was believed that using this particular mixed-methods approach allowed triangulation by examining corroboration between qualitative and quantitative data, and allowing for greater validity of the findings. The specific details given by individuals contributed to meaningful recommendations for the clinic.
- Providing clarity about the purpose of using a mixed-methods protocol will go some way to alleviating the criticisms sometimes levelled at it. For example, you need to be clear about the order in which you conduct your study – for example, if you want to use qualitative data to help clarify results, then the sequence of events should be a survey followed by interviews. Similarly, stating how you plan to integrate your quantitative and qualitative data is a vital step in data analysis (see Chapter 6).
- The student undertaking this project was particularly diligent in their data collection processes, making telephone calls to all potential participants who had received an invitation to complete the survey to prompt them to respond. This can be a rather dispiriting experience with a poor return on effort. However, in the end the survey response rate climbed to 32 per cent (61 out of 192 approached), which was acceptable for this study. The survey fatigue mentioned earlier in this chapter markedly reduces the completion rate for all types of surveys and questionnaires, and it may be that these sorts of actions are required.

Secondary data collection

The data collection methods we have discussed so far have focused on the collection of 'new' data for your project. However, there is also the possibility of using, or more accurately re-using, pre-existing datasets as the source of information for your study. In particular, secondary analysis of statistical datasets is well established. More recently, there has been a push to re-use or re-purpose qualitative datasets, such as researchers' field notes, interview transcripts and observations. There is an ethical component to this: as you will not be inconveniencing people to contribute to a study or project in order to generate new data, as this is already available, you will not be duplicating prior work.

There are various datasets held by institutions and organisations, some of which provide open access to researchers, and so offer a potentially valuable source of data for your study. Knowing what datasets might be available to you can be the first issue. In the UK, Health Data Research UK offers a gateway portal for identifying and applying for some health data (see https://www.hdruk.ac.uk/access-to-health-data/health-data-research-gateway/). And again in the UK, national digital transformation programmes have established regional networks of secure data environments that hold datasets defined by categories such as genomics, maternity community and mental health. Researchers can apply to access the data, but be aware that the legal and governance aspects may be complex and access may take months to organise. A further resource is the UK Data Service, which is the main repository for economic, population and social research data (also in the UK) and can be accessed at: https://ukdataservice.ac.uk/find-data/

Perhaps more practical and easily accessible if you are doing a small or shorter-term project is to identify any local organisations, hospitals or universities, including your own institution, that are likely to have repositories for open-access data. You may be able to use this for your purpose, as the analysis of research data collected previously for another project (with a different aim) is also secondary analysis. Local contacts or other individuals in your networks may allow you access to their data for your project.

The example we use here (Senek et al. 2020) of secondary data collection methods was part of a large dataset of responses to a national employment survey conducted by the Royal College of Nursing (RCN). The anonymous responses to certain items in the survey that had not been included in the overall RCN analysis were analysed as secondary data and used to address a particular aspect of working practices.

Box 5.14: Example of a project using secondary data collection

Title: The Association between Care Left Undone and Temporary Nursing staff Ratios in Acute Settings: A Cross-sectional Survey of Registered Nurses

Background: Previous research has examined understaffing of nurses and found that sub-optimal numbers of registered nurses may result in 'care left undone' and adverse patient outcomes. UK health service providers are increasingly relying on temporary staff to fill permanent posts and this study sought to explore the association between types of nursing staff (temporary or permanent) and quality of care.

Methods: A cross-sectional study analysing the prevalence of self-reported 'care left undone' and staffing resources. It examined the association between staffing levels, proportions of permanent and agency nursing staff, and prevalence of 'care left undone' in adult acute settings.

Data collection: This was a secondary analysis of existing data. The source of data was an online survey of registered nurses (RNs) developed and administered by the Royal College of Nursing (RCN) in 2017 in all four countries that make up the UK. Data was collected between 14 and 30 May 2017. The survey was administered via email and social media and was open to both members and non-members of the RCN. A data-sharing agreement was made between the University of Sheffield and the RCN. The RCN-administered survey was then shared with a research team within the University of Sheffield. All data was anonymised prior to being shared.

Measured outcomes: Data was used to determine the staffing levels and RN agency ratio outcomes (staffing measure) and 'care left undone' measures. These were derived from the responses of 8,841 registered nurses across the UK.

The binary outcome of 'care left undone' was based on respondents' rating of the quality of care provided on their last shift. Respondents rated the statement: *Due to the lack of time, I had to leave necessary care undone* on a 5-point scale *(strongly agree, agree, neither agree nor disagree, disagree, and strongly disagree).* 'Necessary care left undone' was noted to have occurred where the response was 'agree' or 'strongly agree'. To clarify whether there was or was not care left undone, this scale was made into a binary outcome. The middle option on the Likert Scale 'neither agree nor disagree' was treated as a 'missing value'. Data was also available and used to determine the staffing levels and RN agency ratio outcomes (staffing as a ratio of RN present to RN planned, and RN agency staff as a proportion of the RN staff present within a reported shift).

Points to consider:

- Choosing to use secondary sources of data for your study can be a good option; datasets can be large (larger than you might feasibly be able to collect by yourself with your limited budget and time scale). However, there are quite a few governance hurdles to overcome when accessing this type of data, which you must negotiate in plenty of time before committing to secondary data collection as your chosen method.
- A further caution is that your purpose in using and analysing the data will be different to when it was originally collected, and therefore it may not completely meet your needs. Qualitative data is dependent on how it is produced and by whom, meaning subjectivity will affect the construction of the questions asked and available data.
- Finally, as is the case with all retrospective methods of data collection, you will have little opportunity for follow-up or clarification of any data, and it is highly likely that at least some data will be missing.

In Chapter 6 we will discuss how data can be analysed and presented. Then, in Chapter 7 we discuss bringing everything together into a meaningful report and the best ways of communicating your project findings to as wide an audience as possible.

Key points

- The data collection method you employ should align with your overall aims for your project. There is little point in choosing a means of collecting data that you simply cannot do given the scope of your project.
- The main purpose of the data collection should be to obtain data relevant to your project, not just 'nice to know'.
- Use validated and proven sources of data wherever possible, such as validated survey instruments or open-source data, to increase the credibility of your findings.

6

Methods of data analysis

This chapter is concerned with the analysis of your data, which is really about how you come to appreciate and understand it. Making sense of it allows you to develop the 'story' that your data tells, so you can communicate it to others. The way you do this is by drawing on various processes and techniques, which we now discuss.

First, it's worth reiterating here that knowing how you intend to assess the data you collect should be part of the planning stage of the project, outlined in Chapter 3. What is the plan for your data? A common pitfall for experienced and inexperienced researchers alike is to launch into collecting data without having carefully considered what they intend to do with it. A tip here is to keep in mind your study aims and objectives: the goal of your analysis is to provide you with results and/or findings that function to address these. So, rather than simply report everything and anything you find, scrutinise what you report. For example, although compiling tables and graphs describing patients' medical histories would be 'interesting', even if you were able to collect this information with ease, these would largely be irrelevant if your study is about workforce retention. As with all the other steps in your project, the analysis should be rigorous, and carefully and accurately managed (see Box 6.2). However – and this is why data analysis can be so rewarding – the end product will be yours, meaning that you are in charge of it. You have an opportunity to use it to demonstrate to others the significance of what you have found out, and that your interpretation of the data is valid.

Any decisions about what to do with your data will depend in large part on the type of raw data (meaning before you have processed it) you have collected. As with the broad methodological categories set out in Chapter 3, your data will be quantitative or qualitative in nature, although you are likely to have collected some data in both categories.

Basically, quantitative data is numerical in nature, usually in the form of numbers, percentages, categories or measurements rather than words. However, a questionnaire could use words as possible responses – for example, respondents could be asked to choose the word which most describes some aspect of their care, such as 'caring', 'efficient' or 'person-centred'. At first glance this might appear to be qualitative whereas in fact the thing (or variable) that is being measured here is the frequency (the number of times) that each descriptor is selected, making this data numerical. Similarly, while qualitative data is usually in the form of words, or anything else that is not numbers, these data can be quantified and therefore be subject to numerical analysis. The opposite is also true, since quantitative data can also be subject to abstraction and interpretation. The point here is to know and understand the characteristics of the data you want to analyse.

Chapter 5 highlighted various methods of data collection, including: questionnaires, interview recordings, transcripts, charts/records, published documents, diaries, tables, diagrams, computer print outs, field notes, videos and pictures/photographs. A good introduction to the various types of data you might use is the chapter on 'Analysing data' in Blaxter et al. (2010). You are also reminded that the condition of a dataset is unlikely to be perfect because of, for example, illegible handwriting, missing digital records or incomplete files. You will first need to manage the data so that you are able to manipulate it and report on it usefully, a key stage for any type of data analysis.

As suggested above, you need to manage your data well so that you can begin to make sense of it. Data collection (described in Chapter 5) includes deciding on how you intend to record and order the data you collect. For a small-scale project, your data is likely to be gathered into one simple document, such as a spreadsheet, table or transcript. For example, questionnaire responses can be combined into a single document. Some of your data collection sources may be handwritten, such as notebooks, forms or ledgers, but it is likely that your final data document will be digital. It is possible, of course, to perform data analysis 'by hand', but it is uncommon these days.

In this chapter, we illustrate some key approaches to managing and analysing data and provide several examples from projects using widely recognised study designs.

QUANTITATIVE DATA ANALYSIS

Organising your quantitative data for analysis

Using a spreadsheet to record and manage quantitative data, such as Excel or Google Sheets, is a common approach. These types of computer program will be familiar to most researchers, and they are incredibly useful for displaying and manipulating data. However, you should first consider both the nature of your data and how it will be organised for analysis.

If your study uses quantitative data, the analysis will be rooted in mathematical and statistical methods. The choice of which calculation or test you use will be based on the type of data – some analytic procedures, for example, can only be used for data which meet the rules of arithmetic (i.e. data that is of a higher 'level' for analytical purposes). Also, how the data is organised and formatted will be important in enabling the analysis to proceed smoothly.

First of all, you need to decide on the nature of the data – that is, whether it is categorical (nominal or ordinal) or metric (also called interval/ratio level). It is this that will influence which statistical tests you use. As a brief reminder, **categorical** data (the data unit is assigned a category) is considered lower-level data. There are two types of categorical data:

- **Nominal** data is not ordered in any way – for example, blood type is categorised as A, B, AB or O, and has no units of measurement.
- **Ordinal** data, on the other hand, is ordered or ranked, although again it has no units of measurement – for example, students' satisfaction with teaching on a 5-point scale ranging from 'extremely satisfied' to 'extremely dissatisfied'.

Metric (continuous) data, in contrast, is always numerical and gaps between the values can be calculated, examples being body weight or plasma iron levels. Again, there are two types of metric data:

- **Interval** data, when the measurement scale for the data does not include zero – for example, the IQ test has no 'zero' to indicate an absence of intelligence.
- **Ratio** data, when the measurement scale for the data does include zero – this is the highest level of data.

In practice, all metric data can be subjected to the same analytical tests. For a more in-depth treatment, we direct you to Bowers (2020: esp. 34–43), who addresses the fundamental concepts of data and these categories in more depth.

Once you have your data, it will need to be organised further. We call the things being measured 'variables'. For example, 'age' is a variable. How data for this variable is recorded is important as its analysis will be based on mathematical and statistical methods. For example, our age variable will likely be recorded using whole numbers (e.g. 42). Whole numbers lend themselves to most mathematical functions, but if age were recorded in words (e.g. forty-two), arithmetic operations such as addition would be much more difficult and time-consuming. As age is a 'ratio-level' category when recorded as whole numbers (because it is possible to record an age of 0), any statistical test can be used to analyse it. You might also want to group your data into several age categories: 'under 30', '30–49' and 'over 50'. In your spreadsheet, you would record a '1' in the relevant category, based on the age being recorded. Note that the '1' is used here as a code to count frequencies. Similarly, nominal variables that produce values of 'yes/no' are generally coded by replacing 'yes/no' with '0/1'. With this sort of data it would be inappropriate to calculate measures of central tendency, such as the mean.

Grouping together or ordering the data you record will make it easier for you to manage it. Also consider the formatting you use, for example to how many decimal places will you record your data? Variables with missing or unknown data points are usually coded as '9' or '99'. Harnessing the functionality of the programs you use can help you to keep your data accurately. For example, setting rules for formatting (such as not allowing empty cells for certain variables in a spreadsheet, or only accepting numerical data) can aid this. The way that you collect and extract your data in the first place was covered in Chapter 5 (see the data sheet in Figure 5.1), but take time to manage your data during the analysis stage as well.

Data cleaning

This is a process of methodically examining the data you have collected to identify any errors in how it has been coded or recorded in your spreadsheet. This step is often overlooked, but ensuring the data is accurate is vital if you want to confirm the validity of your findings. Ignoring this step might mean your results are inaccurate, and thus potentially damaging, especially if you use your results to make recommendations. The software functionality described above, such as not allowing incomplete data fields, can be a big help here. It is also worth asking a fellow student or colleague to check a sample of your data entries or to work alongside you when entering the data. Common sources of error during data entry include trying to do analysis simultaneously, not entering values for missing data, and trying to do too much in one go when you are tired. For a more detailed look at data-cleaning methods see, for example, Boynton (2017), a key text on data management.

Analysis, interpretation and presentation of quantitative data

Let us now consider the analysis of your data – ordering and transforming so it can be easily understood. Part of this is about presenting it in ways that draw attention to whatever you consider to be particularly important. This is why it is important to put thought into what you plan for your data – the analysis should not merely be the next thing you do after you have collected it. If you have reached this point in your project without yet knowing what you wish to do with the data collected, then you may find yourself in a muddle.

For numerical data this analysis will involve some statistical procedure, and you will need to decide what type of statistics to use. The two main categories are: *descriptive statistics*, used to summarise ('describe') data, and *inferential statistics*, which are used to make comparisons between and inferences about data variables. Conclusions can be drawn using simple descriptive statistics like percentages, averages and proportions, but inferential statistics may be more powerful, such as when testing hypotheses. We discuss both of these approaches in more detail below. However, and as we have stated throughout, we do not intend to explain in detail the processes that make up each aspect of your research project but instead aim to support you in the decisions you make when carrying out your study. For this reason, we urge you to consult key textbooks on research methods which will include chapters on using statistical analysis (e.g. Robson 2024).

You could consider using something more sophisticated than a spreadsheet to analyse your data, especially if using inferential statistics, although this is not always necessary – for example, the popular Statistical Package for the Social Sciences (SPSS). If you think you are out of your depth, seek advice from someone experienced in statistical analysis, although for a small project using a simple study design you are unlikely to be conducting a particularly complicated analysis.

A data analysis plan

It is good practice to create a simple data analysis plan to help focus your analysis on your research question (i.e. list the questions you want answered by the analysis). A plan also helps you with the task of grouping your data appropriately, which is useful for identifying patterns and similarities. Table 6.1 provides an example of an analysis plan, based on the community centre questionnaire study introduced in Chapter 5 (Birch 2024).

Table 6.1 Example analysis plan

Question	Rationale
What is the survey response rate?	To ascertain if results are representative of the population
What are the demographic characteristics of the survey respondents?	To summarise the population accessing the community day centre drop-in sessions Descriptive statistics: categorical data (area, ethnicity, sex) presented as a number and percentage, continuous data (age) presented as the average Addresses the first study aim
How often are respondents using the drop-in sessions? How long for?	Summarises the use of the drop-in centre. Further addresses first aim Descriptive statistics: all data categorical, so presented as a number and percentage
How satisfied are respondents with the drop-in centre?	Descriptive statistics: data are categorical (ordinal) and so presented as frequencies and median Addresses second study aim
Does the gender (sex) or age of respondents correlate to satisfaction scores?	Cross-tabulation of frequencies of variables. (Test depending on numbers of responses, e.g. a chi-squared test with significance set at $p < 0.05$.) Further inference for second study aim
What are the positive and negative aspects of the drop-in centre?	Thematic analysis of long-answer text fields Preliminary codes identified within data to describe content and then patterns and themes identified for reporting

Descriptive statistics

Descriptive statistics do just what the label implies, which is to describe or summarise your data. Although these methods are quite simple, the way that you choose to display and summarise your data can be extremely powerful. Conclusions may be drawn from descriptive statistics, and may be appropriate for the purposes of your project.

Although you will have started with a data plan, you may also have some intuition about what the data is 'telling' you, and you will start to think more about presenting it. A starting place can be spending a bit of time playing with your dataset to explore your first thoughts or hunches to see if your ideas are sound. You could, for example, tabulate your data, possibly using the simplest aspect, which is the frequency (count) of responses (the term 'response' here also indicates numbers of observations/measurements).

A frequency table could be developed for the categories of people who have used a particular service, providing at a glance information about service users. You might decide a graph would show the same information even more clearly, maybe a pie chart to show the proportions (percentages) of people in each category. Or you could use a bar graph to show the range of responses to a Likert-type scale question about 'enjoyment of a course'. Table 6.2 and Figure 6.1 are a frequency table and pie chart respectively showing the ethnicity of participants.

Table 6.2 Frequency table showing the ethnicity of participants

How would you describe your ethnicity?	No. of responses (*n* = 688)	% of total
White (English, Irish, Welsh, Scottish, Gypsy, other white background)	580	84.3
Asian (Indian, Pakistani, Bangladeshi, Chinese, other Asian background)	59	8.6
Black (African, Caribbean, other Black background)	30	4.4
Mixed or multiple ethnic groups	18	2.3
Other	3	0.4

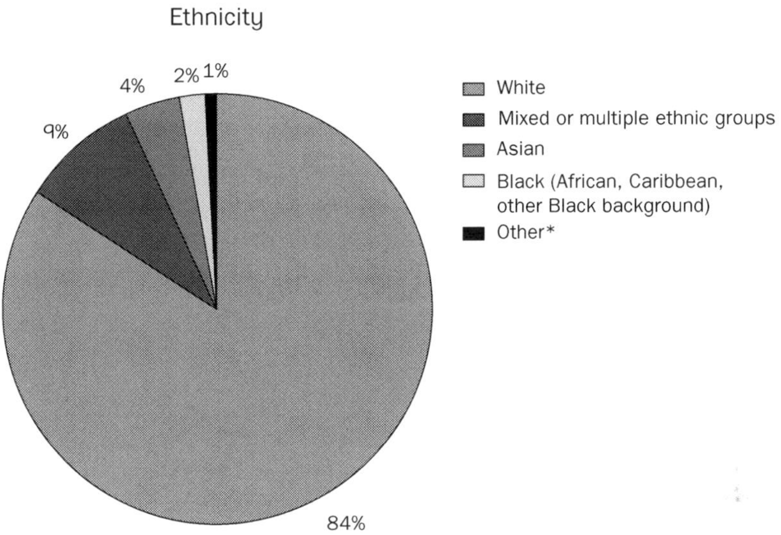

Figure 6.1 Pie chart showing the ethnicity of participants.

A very common form of survey question is to use a scale to find out about the strength of feeling or attitude of respondents, as discussed in Chapter 5. Again, this data could be presented as a table or bar chart (see Table 6.3 and Figure 6.2). It is clear from both that most of the students are confident about their venepuncture skills, but you might have wanted to investigate this further by investigating if the students who are under-confident regarding this skill share any characteristics, or why. If you have the appropriate data, then you might apply some other analysis to investigate this.

Table 6.3 Students' level of confidence in their venepuncture skills

Which statement best describes how confident you are at obtaining a blood sample (venepuncture)?	No. of responses (n = 95)	%
Very confident	30	31.6
Quite confident	56	58.9
Unsure	8	8.4
Extremely unconfident	1	1.1

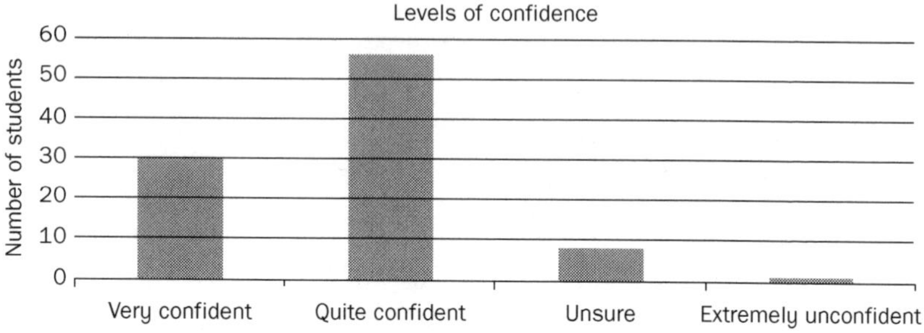

Figure 6.2 Bar chart showing students' level of confidence in their venepuncture skills.

Descriptive statistics of central tendency are used to demonstrate 'the most typical' value of a dataset, what most of us call the 'average'. There are three ways of calculating this, based on the underlying characteristics of the data. The mean, which is the arithmetic average, should really only be used to calculate data with full mathematical properties. The mode, the value that occurs most often within the dataset, is appropriate with nominal data, while the median (or mid-score) may be used for calculation if extreme values are present (although it should not be used for nominal data).

The bar chart shown in Figure 6.3 clearly shows that the 'average' (or most common) number of appointments for the respondents to this survey was two. The average described here is the mode (the most frequent response); using the mean would not be appropriate as 'number of appointments' is a categorical value.

Additional information about the variability of data can be provided by looking at the spread of the data (or dispersion) around the central tendency; the measures used are range, semi-interquartile range and standard deviation. The standard deviation (SD) is commonly reported along with mean values, and the semi-interquartile range with median values.

In another project, we looked at the ages of patients attending a clinic. Their mean age was 34 years, with a standard deviation of 5.73. Now while this standard deviation is fairly small, variability in data is most useful when comparing two sets of findings (e.g. if we decided to look at the spread of ages for patients in clinics from different locations).

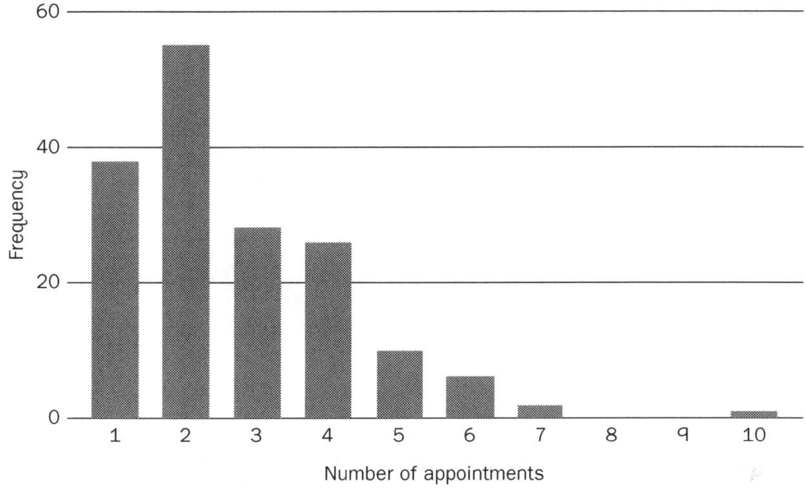

Figure 6.3 A bar chart of number of appointments.

An important statistical concept related to the spread of data around the central tendency is normal distribution (see Figure 6.4). This is the assumption that many human properties, such as test scores, IQ and weight are close to the mean value. When this is plotted on a graph, the values follow a 'bell curve' – which means the majority of scores are in the middle area (68% within 1 SD and 95% within 2 SD), and very few people would have scores on either side of the majority. Many statistical decisions are based on an assumption that data follow this distribution. When using inferential statistics, you should estimate if this is the case for your data as the selection of statistical tests used will be dependent on this.

If you are using descriptive statistics to analyse non-categorical data, then a graphical representation of average values for properties can be useful. For example, the weight and BMI graphs of patients attending a clinic in a student service evaluation project is shown in Figure 6.5. The distribution is not a bell curve, but rather skewed, meaning on average being heavier compared with the general population. However, note that because the sample size was small, we cannot be confident that assumptions about this cohort can be transferable to other populations.

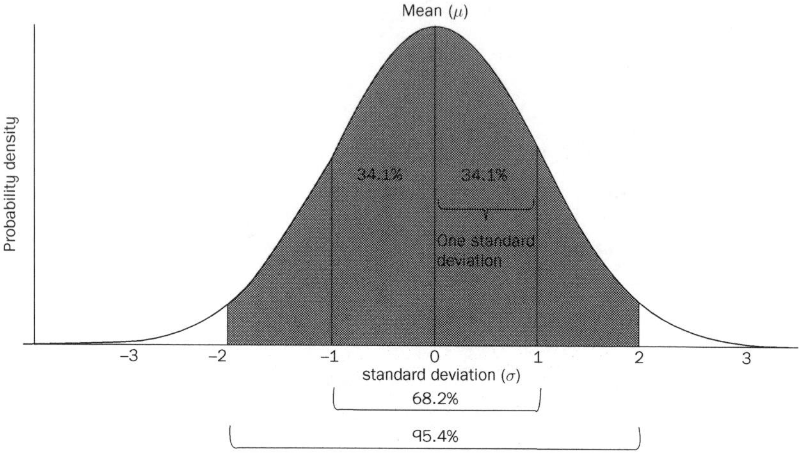

Figure 6.4 Standard deviation from the mean of normal distribution.

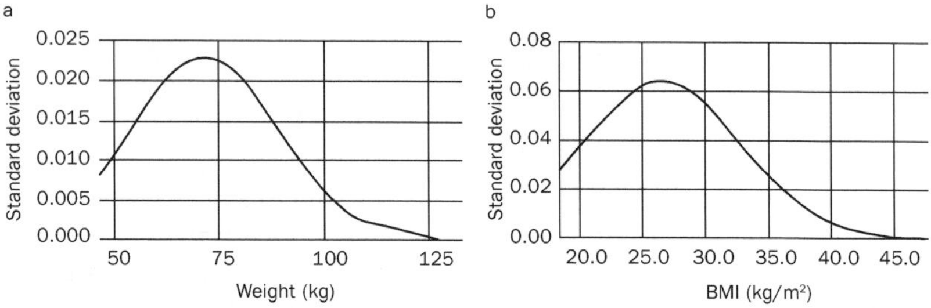

Figure 6.5 Graphs showing ranges of weight and BMI of patients in a clinic.

Inferential statistics

These are statistical tests that make inferences (estimates or predictions) about relationships (correlations) between variables or groups in the sample, and whether these inferences can be generalised to the wider population of interest. There are specific tests depending on what you are looking for. For many, much like the measures of central tendency we looked at earlier, this choice will depend on the type of data (categorical and so on) and the amount of data you have. Metric data, which are normally distributed, can be analysed with the more powerful parametric tests, such as t-tests and analysis of variance (ANOVA). Non-parametric tests, which are less powerful, are used for categorical data, or data that is not normally distributed. The most common example of a non-parametric test is the chi-squared statistic (χ^2), which is used to look for differences in the expected and observed frequencies (counts) of groups of data. A way of examining this is with cross-tabulation, whereby tables of results for one answer are compared with those for another answer, for example levels of satisfaction with a service against the gender of respondents.

Other common correlation tests are Spearman's rank correlation (rho) (for ordinal data) and Pearson (r) (metric data). These calculate a correlation coefficient which will always be a value between +1 and −1. This indicates the strength of the relationship between two variables. If the relationship is positive, then as one variable increases so does the other (e.g. height and weight), whereas if it is negative, as one variable increases the other reduces (attendance at school and student marks). A correlation coefficient near zero indicates hardly any relationship at all. Tests for interrelationships between three or more variables, such as multiple regression, use multivariate statistics. Again, we urge you to seek guidance when deciding which tests to use for data analysis in your project.

All statistical tests of correlation report the results as a test statistic, usually in the form of a letter (such as U for the Mann-Whitney test). How significant the results of each test are will be shown by its probability value (p) – how likely the results of the sample would have happened by chance. Test results with a value of $p < 0.05$ are considered to be statistically significant; there is a less than 5 per cent chance that the results would have happened by chance alone. Other levels of probability often reported are $p < 0.01$ (1%) and $p < 0.001$ (0.01%), but in most cases a 5 per cent value is acceptable. Results which fail to reach significance are labelled 'ns', or non-significant. Confidence intervals (CIs) are also used to assess statistical significance. They are the range of values within which we can be confident contains the true value for a (general) population. These are generally set at 95 per cent. Statistical calculation will provide a point estimate for the data sample; if this lies outside the CIs, then it is not statistically significant. This also indicates precision of results; the wider the CIs, the less accurate the estimated results will be.

Importantly, statistically significant results do not necessarily tell you that your study has found out something important. It would be just as interesting to find that there are no significant relationships in your data sample. Various errors can be made during statistical analysis, when the wrong or poor conclusions are drawn from the results; these are known as type I and type II errors – again, frequently due to poor sample sizes. Furthermore, there are other statistical measures of clinical significance, usually undertaken in epidemiological studies that seek to estimate health risks and treatment outcomes in populations – studies that will be much larger than the types of projects covered in this book. These include odds ratios and relative risk. We advise that you read more widely, including the excellent chapter by Peat (2001) and the text by Harris and Taylor (2021). Box 6.1 is a snapshot of a study conducted by Imms (2025).

Box 6.1: Service evaluation of a ventricular tachycardia clinic using quantitative techniques

Title: A Service Evaluation of a Nurse-led, Fast-track Ventricular Tachycardia Clinic

Background: Cardiac implantable electronic defibrillators (CIEDs) are crucial for managing heart failure and preventing arrhythmic death. Around 23 per cent of patients fitted with these devices (e.g. pacemakers) receive CIED therapy (internal shock and anti-tachycardia (ATP) pacing) in response to cardiac events (ventricular arrhythmia) within 3 years, which can have significant clinical and psychological impacts. There is an absence of structured pathways for patients receiving CIED therapy. In response, a fast-track, nurse-led ventricular tachycardia clinic was established to offer early review, device optimisation and treatment escalation.

Aim: To evaluate clinical outcomes for CIED patients following early intervention at the nurse-led ventricular tachycardia clinic for patients undergoing CIED therapy.

Objectives: (1) To determine whether device therapy decreases following clinic interventions (procedural and/or medication-related). (2) To assess whether hospital admissions for ventricular tachycardia decline after clinic intervention.

Methods: A service evaluation of 88 participants (2022–24) reviewed electronic records, documented interventions, and measured therapy burden at baseline and 6 months. The sample size was justified given the newness of the service and practical constraints.

Specific outcomes measured included device therapy burden, clinic interventions, and service wait times. A robust comparative analysis of outcomes (device therapy burden) before and after clinic intervention was undertaken.

Outcomes were assessed at 6 months post-intervention (clinic admission) by reviewing arrhythmia burden, subsequent therapy, and hospital admissions, using electronic care records and remote monitoring systems.

Results: There was a significant reduction ($p < 0.01$) in CIED therapy (shock vs. anti-tachycardia pacing [ATP] therapy) and hospitalisations at 6 months for patients receiving early intervention at the fast-track, nurse-led VT clinic.

The data gathered by Imms (2025) were initially categorised as numerical or categorical variables. Numerical data were assessed for normality via histogram inspection. Parametric data were summarised using the mean and standard deviation, while non-parametric data were reported using the median and interquartile range (IQR) to account for any skewness. Categorical variables, such as gender and aetiology, were summarised as counts and percentages.

Comparisons between two groups (shock vs. ATP therapy) for numerical data used independent t-tests for parametric variables, with significance set at $p < 0.05$, while non-parametric comparisons used the Wilcoxon rank-sum test where appropriate (age, left ventricular ejection fraction, and therapy counts). Categorical comparisons employed the chi-square test. Paired data within groups (e.g. changes in therapy burden from baseline to 6 months) were analysed using the Wilcoxon signed-rank test. All statistical analyses were conducted using R version 4.4.0.

Selected results following analysis are as follows:

Hospitalisation as part of index presentation

Hospitalisation was assessed across the sample ($n = 87$) and therapy groups (see Figure 6.6). Overall, 37 per cent ($n = 32$) attended hospital at initial presentation: 25 per cent ($n = 10$) in the ATP group and 46 per cent ($n = 22$) in the shock group. Although the difference was not statistically significant ($p = 0.06$), hospitalisation was more frequent in the shock group.

Clinical waiting time

Clinic wait time demonstrated a mean of 11 days, with a standard deviation of 13 days. Figure 6.7 shows the distribution of waiting list times; most participants were seen in clinic within 10 days.

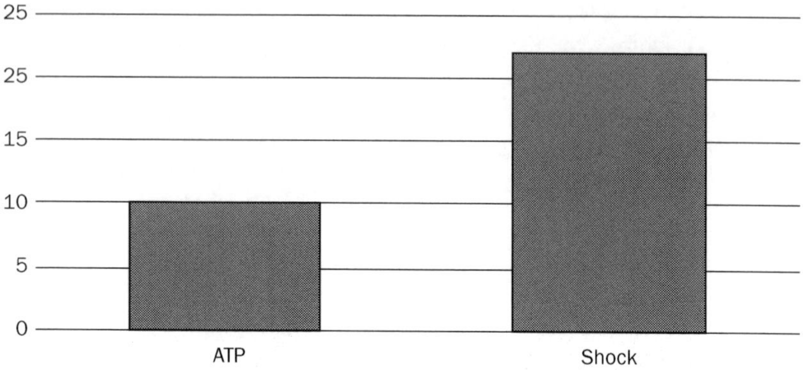

Figure 6.6 Hospitalisation at presentation.

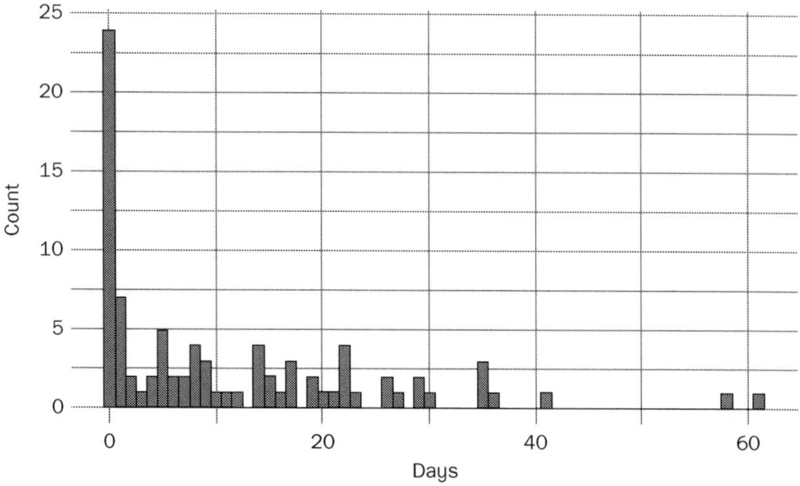

Figure 6.7 Distribution of waiting list times.

Waiting times were compared between groups: for the ATP group (n = 40) there was a median of 8.5 days (IQR 19.5), and for the shock group (n = 47) 5 days (IQR 14.5) (see Figure 6.8). Shock participants were reviewed sooner, but the difference was not statistically significant (p = 0.5).

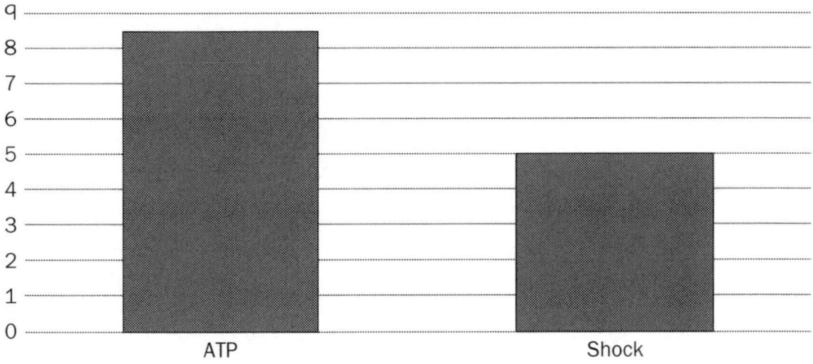

Figure 6.8 Waiting times – shock vs. ATP therapy.

Medications by presenting therapy: dose adjustments or initiated heart failure medication

Figure 6.9 shows dose adjustments and initiated medications as a percentage and split by subgroup: ATP (n = 40) and shock (n = 47). This demonstrates increased intervention or titration in the ATP group, aside from mineralocorticoid receptor antagonists (MRAs). However, this was not statistically significant ($p > 0.05$).

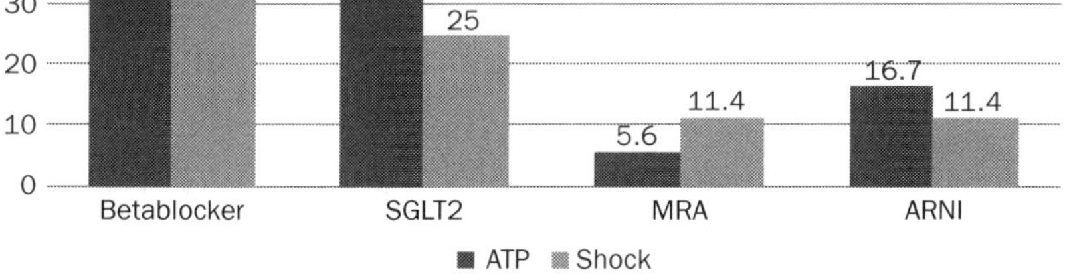

Figure 6.9 Dose adjustments vs. initiated medications.

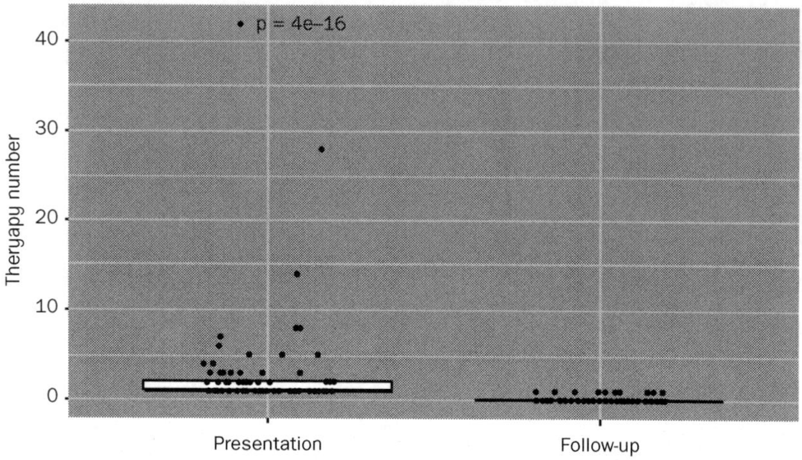

Figure 6.10 Therapy numbers at presentation and at 6 months follow-up.

Overall therapy numbers at presentation and at 6 months follow-up

The box plot in Figure 6.10 demonstrates a reduction in overall therapy shock and ATP from presentation to 6 months follow-up. This was statistically significant $p < 0.01$.

Concepts of quality

There are several ways in which the overall quality of your research project can be judged. As noted in Chapter 2, an assessment can be made using a critical appraisal tool (see, for example, the Critical Appraisal Skills Programme: https://casp-uk.net/casp-tools-checklists/) or reporting guidelines (e.g. https://www.equator-network.org/reporting-guidelines/). Good practice is to consider them in relation to your own study. Many are to do with the overall approach but are particularly relevant to your analysis of data and interpretation of results. When you are introducing your findings to others, you will want to know that your work merits their time and attention; you will be more confident about this if you also trust your own work. See Box 6.2 for some of the main criteria for judging the quality of projects.

Box 6.2: How to assess quality

Reliability is a term most often used for quantitative methods and indicates the extent to which the results obtained would be reproduced if the same study were repeated by another researcher – that is, how consistent, dependable and repeatable the results would be.

Validity is also relevant in quantitative studies – this is whether the tool you have used measures whatever it is you set out to measure. So, although your results might be repeated if you did the study many times, if they don't tell you want you are trying to find out, then they would not be valid. Accuracy in collecting and reporting data is also important here, as is use of appropriate sampling methods (recall how inferential statistics assume samples are representative).

Bias can distort results or study findings. Bias might relate to the sample (or participants) being atypical owing to its composition or poor recruitment. This is why the inclusion/exclusion criteria must be clearly stated if the sample is a group. Qualitative studies must also show clearly decisions made about who was included – individuals with appropriate experience and a variety of social affiliations. The study may have transferability to other settings; this may be indicated by findings which resonate with existing evidence or with readers.

Rigour is a more general concept about how the whole study was approached and designed. Rigour will be demonstrated by you being systematic, consistent and accurate during each stage of the project. It also means paying attention to – and being transparent about – things that may negatively influence the study findings. This includes recognising any limitations with the study design and outlining any steps taken to address them. It is far better if you highlight these, as it will show that you understand what you have done and that you have the knowledge to perhaps do better.

For further reading, see Heale and Twycross (2015), Kuper et al. (2008) and Barbour (2014).

QUALITATIVE DATA ANALYSIS

Organising your qualitative data for analysis

Just as numerical data needs to be managed and organised before your analysis 'proper' can begin, the same applies to raw qualitative data. For the purposes of this book, we use qualitative to mean data in the form of words, although other documentary sources such as pictures can also be used in qualitative analysis. Generally, the words you have gathered as your data will have come from spoken or written survey responses (e.g. as answers to open-ended questions or interviews).

Spoken data, such as that recorded in an interview, will need to be transcribed. Until recently, this was a question of listening to the recording that you made and writing down – or typing out – what was said or employing another person to do this for you. Nowadays transcribing is a far easier process and there are many applications that will do this – at least partially – for you. For example, most recordings of online meetings can be directed to make a transcript available. You will, however, need to listen to the recording yourself and check it against the transcript generated (however it is produced) because it will need to be refined before use. Furthermore, you need to make yourself familiar with the interview itself, not just the words spoken, but how they were spoken and the length of any silences, as this will aid your understanding of the data. Also be aware that the quality of recordings can vary, so you may have to listen to them several times to confirm what has been said.

You will want to keep your written data in one place. Where this is will depend on your approach but it might be in standard electronic format (such as Microsoft Word) or by using software such as ATLAS Ti or NVivo. Some researchers print their transcriptions out and do much of their manipulation and organisation of the data 'by hand', but most will use some sort of electronic format to store the data for their study. That way they can manage it (sorting, coding, selecting, labelling and summarising) easily.

The data-cleaning principles that we introduced for qualitative data are similarly important here, although perhaps you will approach it in a less mechanical way. The words that you have in text form should absolutely be the accurate account of what was said (or written in reply as an answer to a question), so this data should be checked to confirm this is the case, including things like checking for missing data such as text responses to survey questions and, as above, that the transcription is correct.

Analysis, interpretation and presentation of qualitative data

Qualitative data analysis might appear to you to be very different to the rules, statistics and arithmetic used in numerical data analysis, but the purpose remains the same (to make sense of and present the data). At its most basic, qualitative approaches seek to ascribe meanings to what has been said (or written). Usually this is by identifying and assigning meaning to patterns and themes.

It has been said that the subjectivity inherent in qualitative analysis (meaning the interpretation of the data by the person analysing it) makes it less rigorous. This is why you must take a systematic and evidence-based approach to your qualitative analysis (for more on rigour, see Box 6.2).

In Chapter 3, we highlighted that the tradition of qualitative study includes several theoretical approaches, and that if you are undertaking a larger study, you might be strongly wedded to one of these, for example phenomenology, grounded theory or ethnography. For a critical appraisal of these and other methods, see Aveyard et al. (2026). If you choose to use one of these approaches to data analysis, consult the relevant authoritative sources. However, as readers of this book we anticipate your approach will be more generalist, and as such we provide a broad overview of the two most widely used approaches to qualitative analysis in small-scale projects: thematic analysis and content analysis.

Thematic analysis

There are two main approaches to thematic analysis: reflexive thematic analysis (RTA; Braun and Clarke 2022), which is a flexible, interpretative approach to qualitative data, and the Framework Method (Gale et al. 2013), which is a more structured and systematic method, especially suited for large, applied studies. Although both approaches are suitable for analysing qualitative data, they differ in the way that you will go about the process.

The most well-known source for reflective thematic analysis is Braun and Clarke (2022), who describe thematic analysis as 'a method for identifying, analysing and reporting patterns (themes) within data' (2022: 4) using the six-stage model described below (with our commentary).

Phase 1: Becoming familiar with the data. This is where you read and re-read the transcripts so that you have a thorough understanding of each interview you conducted. As mentioned above, software can aid you in this, but it is not a substitute for a thorough reading of the scripts.

Phase 2: Creating initial codes. This is where you attach some initial meaning to your interview data. These are tentative and are likely to change as your analysis continues but they are important as a launch pad to get you started with the analysis.

Phase 3: Searching for themes. As you develop initial themes, you will see patterns emerge. These remain tentative at this stage, but a picture will begin to take shape.
Phase 4: Reviewing themes. Developing themes will be an iterative process as you work through the complete dataset. The themes will become stronger as you continue to code the interviews. Codes which initially looked strong might appear less meaningful as you progress with the analysis or vice versa.
Phase 5: Defining and naming themes. This is the final phase of the analysis, where you name each theme and the codes within it. Note that this is very similar to constant comparative analysis, which requires the continual 'dynamic working back and forth' (Lincoln and Guba 1985: 342) of examining and coding data until a robust dataset is established.
Phase 6: Producing the report. This is the final write-up of the project where you commit to the dataset you have established.

Braun and Clarke (2022) remind us of the importance of using the appropriate selective data (in the form of data extracts, quotations) to convincingly illustrate the validity of an analysis. This goes further than merely describing data patterns; the interpretation should relate to understanding data in relation to the research question.

Box 6.3 provides an example of thematic analysis, adapted from Widdows (2022).

Box 6.3: Example of findings using qualitative reflective thematic analysis

One section of findings for this service evaluation project was the thematic analysis of interviews.

Two major themes emerged from the data collected. Theme one was 'pressure of decision-making', which reflected thoughts surrounding the initial appeal of intrauterine conception (IUC) as well as the effectiveness and timing of the information received prior to insertion at the clinic.

4.2.1: Pressure of decision-making. This theme included various sub-themes: 'appeal of intrauterine contraception', 'effectiveness of information' and 'timing'.

4.2.1.1: Appeal of intrauterine contraception. *When discussing the use of a coil, many participants explored their reasons for considering IUC.*

Here women explored ideas about their previous contraceptive experiences, effectiveness of IUC, and perceptions of ease. Women considered the benefits of IUC in relation to other contraceptives they might have used, perceiving it to be 'easier than taking the pill'. IUC was also seen as a more flexible alternative to tubal ligation: 'The other extreme was the sterilisation was just … I was taking the choice away completely'. Some survey participants cited that they 'had the coil previously and liked it'. These women reported that they 'knew it worked' and therefore expressed confidence in the coil: 'I'd had the coil before and I don't want any more babies'; 'Had one before, works well'. Participants opting for the copper coil 'liked the fact there were no hormones', in contrast to other largely hormonal contraception available to them. 'I knew that it wasn't hormonal so that was a big benefit to me because I'd had some struggles with hormonal contraception'.

Framework analysis, as discussed by Gale et al. (2013), is an alternative to thematic analysis. This method is like reflective thematic analysis, but data is analysed within a framework, either one that is external to the project or one that is derived from initial thematic analysis. For a detailed example of framework analysis, we suggest you consult the paper by Arifin et al. (2021), where the method is used in a midwifery research project.

Content analysis

Content analysis is perhaps most suitable for the analysis of longer text answers collected by questionnaires. This is a systematic technique where data is grouped into simple themes (codes), often based on words or phrases which are repeated across multiple responses to the same question, and then the frequency of themes is counted and discussed in relation to the overall study aim. Themes that occur frequently are considered worthy of further investigation and for confirmation of other findings, such as further explanation of numerical results from the same study.

One part of the findings from the service evaluation project by Widdows was a content analysis of the free-text survey question about why participants had chosen intrauterine contraception (see Table 6.4, adapted from Widdows 2022).

Table 6.4 Example of findings using qualitative content analysis

Code	Incidence
Advised by healthcare professional	9
Avoiding other contraceptives	13
Convenient	18
Effective	4
Family complete	7
Immediate contraception	2
Long-acting	11
No periods	2
Non-hormonal	8

In summary, you need to identify the approach to data analysis that meets the needs of your project, and you must justify its choice. Your data analysis enables you to be creative – be bold and confident if you can justify your approach. Your overall results or findings should always relate back to your project aim – do not forget to address your research question when you report your findings/results. For example, if you have undertaken an audit, do the results suggest that the standard you were measuring against was reached? Does your service evaluation clearly show what level the service is performing at, and how do you know this? For small-scale research projects, do you have a clear statement of findings which answer your research question?

Bringing it together: synthesis

The final part of data analysis is to bring everything together into a coherent whole; this is sometimes referred to as synthesis. However, the terms synthesis and analysis are often used interchangeably. To keep things simple, we will use the term synthesis for when you have two datasets, for example from mixed methods, and you need to integrate the two: whether this is descriptive and inferential statistical analysis or the presentation of a thematic or content analysis.

If you are combining two types of results, for example from a mixed-methods study, then you need to include an extra step that shows how you integrated the findings from the two. Creswell and Plano Clark (2018) provide detailed guidance for this. In a nutshell, the sequence you undertake involves one of three options:

1. Quantitative findings are shown to be explained by the qualitative results ('explanatory'). This approach is undertaken when there is sufficient knowledge about a topic to devise a questionnaire, whose results are then explored in a qualitative study.
2. Qualitative findings are followed by quantitative findings in order to confirm the commonality of issues ('exploratory'). This approach is undertaken when there is insufficient understanding about a topic and qualitative data is required in order to obtain this.
3. The two analyses are undertaken simultaneously ('convergent'). This approach is undertaken where there is no clear need for one type of data over another.

The challenge in the presentation of data in a mixed-methods project is to avoid repetition as different data sources are likely to convey similar findings or results. You will need to discuss with your supervisor how to present your data so as to avoid repetition but at the same time to demonstrate the breadth and complexity of the data you have collected and analysed. For example, the final synthesis of a mixed-methods project might be the presentation of themes incorporating the quantitative data into the thematic analysis.

In the next chapter, we look at the final stage of your study journey, which is the writing up and dissemination of your work.

Key points

- Data analysis should be undertaken in a systematic and accurate way.
- The analysis starts with managing and understanding the raw data before undertaking any other steps in the process.
- Quantitative (numerical) data are analysed by methods of descriptive and inferential statistics.
- Qualitative (words) data analysis seeks to make sense of what people have said, often by searching for patterns and meanings in the data.
- The final part of data analysis is to make a persuasive case for the story that the data is telling.

7

Writing up and dissemination

At this stage in your project, you have identified your question and provided rationale for it and the project itself, used relevant data collection methods, analysed your data and decided how to present it. Now it is time to write up your findings. We suggest that you write up each chapter as you complete it: Introduction, Background, Literature Review, Methods, Results/Findings, Discussion (see our reporting guideline at the end of this chapter). We also suggest that you pause once you have completed your results/findings. This represents a natural break in your work; you have collected and analysed your data and the next step is to decide what it means. Take your time and remember that you cannot start your discussion section until you have completed your results/findings, as the former is linked to the latter.

Articulating the ideas generated by your study forms the 'discussion' section; it is an often-overlooked activity, undertaken at the end of the project when energy levels are low and you are unsure of what to include. However, it is a key section of the write up, and doing it well allows you to subsequently make solid conclusions and recommendations, thus bringing the project to a successful close.

The aim of the discussion section is to explain what your findings/results mean in relation to your research question, other research, theories or policy. You should also reflect and think about whether your question has been answered. Consider the judicious use of artificial intelligence (AI) (refer to Box 1.2 on page 21) for small tasks such as checking sentence structure and grammar or identifying alternative words. Do not be tempted to use AI more extensively as not only will you be in breach of your institution's regulations, you are likely to find that it doesn't offer a true representation of the ideas you wish to portray.

How to write your discussion

Remember, your discussion should not be a repeat of your results/findings – it is an opportunity to tell the reader what your findings really mean. You began your project because you wanted to solve a practice dilemma or find out more about a particular clinical problem, so the discussion section is where you bring everything together by explaining what your results mean and how they relate to your chosen question and other research. You are now free to express your own opinions but remember to use supporting evidence or literature from your introduction/background sections. Also, you may want to compare your findings against national or local standards, policy documents or guidelines.

Some people are more comfortable adhering to a structure for their discussion. Watson (2018), for example, has suggested a series of steps you could follow. He recommends you start by paraphrasing the aims and the research question and then reiterating – albeit briefly – what the results show. Although someone reading your work will have already read the results/findings section, a clearly articulated summary is always useful here. This might take a few drafts to get right, so consider asking someone who has not been involved in your study to review it so that you get another perspective on what you have written.

Once you have a few sentences that accurately reflect your findings, you can move onto the main part of the discussion. You will want to use the results of your analysis (your findings) to explain why things are as you have found them to be, and show you understand the issues or questions that have arisen. To do this, you can go through the results in turn, relating them to other relevant research, theory or policy and providing a commentary on what you think this reveals. For example, if there are research findings in a related area, that are similar or dissimilar to yours, you can draw on these. If your findings reflect a particular theory, you can introduce that theory here. If you have identified a theory to explain why some people behave the way they do, then state what this is. Similarly, if there is a policy that either supports your findings or indeed seems to contradict them, draw on it. The important thing is that you move the discussion away from your findings and towards broader concepts to which your findings point. On a practical note, try not to refer to any findings in your discussion; instead, you need to focus on the bigger picture. For example, in a master's study undertaken with several MSc students, Aveyard et al. (2022) explored how nurses provide information to patients prior to nursing care procedures. Findings identified that information was given in a consistent manner and that every nurse interviewed was committed to the principle that the patient should be informed about their care. However, the focus of the information-giving was to inform rather than to facilitate informed consent. In the discussion, these findings were summarised concisely and then used as a springboard to discuss how information-giving as a means to inform the patient about what is going to happen is different from the concept of informed consent – where information is given as part of a process that facilitates the patient's involvement in the decision-making process.

Don't forget to comment on whether you believe the aims of the project were addressed and whether the research question was answered. For someone undertaking an audit, this will require making a statement about whether the national standard has indeed been met and what further action needs to be taken. For those of you undertaking a service evaluation, you should also discuss the next steps in the cycle of service improvement.

You also need to discuss any limitations to your project or its findings. One limitation might relate to how early interviews were conducted, but how your skill in this endeavour developed as you proceeded. A further limitation might relate to questionnaire design or how it was piloted. As a general rule, reflect on the method you used and consider how you might have done things differently if you had more time, resources and indeed the benefit of hindsight. Whilst you should be honest about any limitations and how you would overcome them in the future, do not dwell on them; instead, let the discussion highlight the positives of your project.

You are now ready to write the final sections of your dissertation: (1) your conclusions and (2) any recommendations and implications for future practice. Once again you will be expected to make a final – though very short – summary of the findings and refer back to your research question and state whether you think it was addressed successfully. At this stage, do not introduce any new literature or data.

It is now time to make recommendations and highlight any implications for future practice or research. This is often done as a bullet point list, which allows you to be thorough but concise – remember that you have a word count to adhere to! Finish this section with a clear but succinct statement or overview about your project. Make sure it feels like you are 'concluding the conclusion'. Ensure your recommendations are an exact fit and can be traced back to the findings. This is not a time to go off at a tangent or step onto your own personal soapbox to have a rant; instead, allow your enthusiasm for your project to shine through in your final remarks, highlighting the contribution you have made to the knowledge base and the benefits you have taken from your research journey.

You will be aware that an audit, service evaluation and small-scale research project will each have their own impact on the world of health care. Audits and service evaluations will have an impact at the local level, as is their intention: their results will feed back into the healthcare cycle of quality improvement, as discussed in Chapter 1. Both types of project are intended for internal, local quality improvement, yet provide quick results that are actionable, so their benefit locally can be significant. The results of a small-scale research project have the potential for generalisation to a wider healthcare setting, although it is important to remember this will be limited due to the size and scope of the project. Therefore, the way the findings from the different projects are reported and disseminated to practitioners, stakeholders and service users will differ.

The next section will explore the different approaches to the dissemination of your findings, and how to reach different target audiences.

Dissemination

Reality check! You might have thought it would be relatively straightforward to disseminate research findings having read all of the above, yet this ignores the fact that your findings could be controversial or critical of current practice. It is not easy to challenge practice and yet the purpose of doing a small-scale research project, of course, is to do exactly that. This somewhat uncomfortable state of affairs has been coined 'cultural suicide', whereby you are excluded by some colleagues and others feel you have betrayed them, a concept introduced by Brookfield (1993) in relation to critical thinking in health care.

An audit or service evaluation will have been conducted on behalf of an organisation and it is therefore reasonable to expect that they will be interested in your findings. This might not be the case for small-scale research where the project won't necessarily be directly linked to a clinical area. In this case, you need to consider how your findings might be received.

Imagine, for example, how you would feel if you were told (or it was implied) that you were 'white centric' or even 'racist' in your educational practice. Oozageer Gunowa et al. (2021) conducted a review of education documentation regarding wound care teaching, as well as interviews and focus groups with students and academic staff in five higher education institutes. She found scant reference to care for people across a range of skin tones within the curriculum and that those interviewed confirmed this was standard practice and a difficult but important message to hear.

So, it is best to be realistic that not all findings will be accepted with open arms by your colleagues or institution; there will be some who will be cautious or even sceptical of the changes you suggest. You need to learn to navigate around these feelings and behaviours exhibited by others towards you and your research. There are resources you can use to help disseminate your work, which we consider in the next section.

Following the review of Oozageer Gunowa et al. (2021), there is general recognition that neither nurse nor medical education (e.g. Hartland and Larkai 2020) should be delivered in a 'white centric' bubble, thus perpetuating a racist culture within health care. This has led to a distinct change in the way that educational materials are developed for the identification of pressure injury for all people, including recommendations for the representation of darker skin tones in simulation-based education. Furthermore, this has led to a wider debate about how issues of inclusivity in education are addressed.

At other times, researchers find that they are pushing at an open door with their findings. For example, Forde-Johnston (2025) explored the impact of the use of electronic patient records on the interaction between nurse and patient. Findings demonstrated that the use of electronic records led to significant changes in the way nurses and patients interacted, with the use of a computer screen leading to an emphasis on closed questions. Dissemination of findings indicated they resonated with colleagues both nationally and internationally. For example, a chief nursing officer commented on social media: 'Your study is really interesting, and I will reflect for some time on how we can rebalance the nurse-patient relationship post-EPR. It's certainly not something I have ever seen considered in EPR rollouts, and it's damage already done that needs fixing'.

Both of the above projects (Oozageer Gunowa et al., 2021; Forde-Johnston 2025) were more large-scale doctoral studies and hence would be expected to have a greater impact than a small-scale project. However, it is important to focus on dissemination – in other words, 'finding your voice': sharing your findings with others, so that your work can influence practice, inform staff or patients, and lead to positive outcomes for individuals and communities. You will also want your findings to be communicated to board members of your organisation, particularly if you are reporting back on the results of an audit or service evaluation, or need to provide justification for the funding of a new initiative or continuing service. For example, in a service evaluation of recognising acute illness and deterioration (RAID) huddles, Abel (2023) reported how, over the study period, they were able to reduce cardiac arrest calls and support the recognition and escalation of clinical deterioration calls. Improved patient outcomes and enhanced patient safety were direct benefits of the RAID huddles and in cases like this, the results deserve to be disseminated as widely as possible.

Making your research count is important because it ensures that the knowledge produced has real value beyond the academic award you may be studying for. It also honours the time and effort of participants and yourself by generating findings that can be applied in meaningful ways. Also, sharing results allows other researchers to build on your work, advancing knowledge in the field. Finally, making research count demonstrates accountability to funders, employers and institutions, while also strengthening your own professional credibility and opportunities. Demonstrating your research experience is increasingly used and welcomed in applications for promotions or new roles, or even in your professional revalidation process.

How can I share my findings?

You can share the findings from your small-scale research project in several ways. From an academic perspective, this might include uploading the work to a university repository, presenting at conferences, displaying study findings as a poster or writing a journal article. Professionally, you can share findings with organisations, practitioners and policy-makers via reports or presentations.

Public options include writing blogs, posting infographics on social media, and giving community talks. You may also work with supervisors to publish or expand the project, or you might decide to use your project as a springboard to a doctoral application or to seek funding for further research.

The method you use will depend on the topic of your project and the audience who will benefit most. Let us now consider the different methods in turn.

Academic output

If you have undertaken your project as an educational endeavour, such as an undergraduate thesis or master's dissertation, you will be looking to make good of the associated academic credit that entails. But this has the associated disadvantage that beyond the markers of your work, its reach will be limited unless you take specific action to raise awareness of your project among the academic and practice community. So, we encourage you to consider one or more of the following options to get your work noticed.

Publication

For those of you undertaking a small-scale research study, you can plan to publish your findings in a relevant journal. This could be a professional journal, an in-house organisational journal, or even a newsletter. In the publication you can acknowledge that one of the limitations of the study was its scope: study at this level is by definition small-scale in nature and the data was likely collected in one or two clinical areas only. For those of you undertaking an audit or service evaluation, publication of your work is less likely – though not impossible if you have received the correct permissions – as the findings relate directly to one clinical area and are not generalisable. However, there are other avenues you can take to disseminate your work such as at conferences and on social media, which we shall discuss next.

Adapting your project findings into a shorter article for peer review is a valuable use of your time, but will require some effort to edit it into the style and length required. You will need to understand what the requirements are of the journal and this can be found under the 'author guidelines' for that particular journal. Try to select one where you feel the readership reflects who you want to inform and engage with. Is it a journal you regularly read and are familiar with? If not, spend some time reading published work from a few issues to get a feel for the style and requirements of the journal. Adapting a longer piece of work for submission to a publication is not as easy as just cutting words out; it takes time to reshape your work and decide what critical information needs to be included and what can be safely omitted. Holland and Watson (2021) provide a guide to the process of publishing within nursing and health care, and will act as a useful resource as you adapt and write your article.

George, for example, undertook a small-scale research project in which he explored how people on a low income accessed primary care services. In this project (see George and Aveyard, 2020) he interviewed attendees at a day centre in order to find out how they did so. These findings were published as a research paper in the *British Journal of Community Nursing*.

Conference presentations – both poster and oral

A great way of getting others to engage with your project and its findings at a local or national level is to submit an abstract to present a poster or short talk at a subject-specific conference or postgraduate research event.

A poster allows you to share key results in a clear, visual format that is easy for others to read quickly. As conferences usually require you to stand by your poster at certain directed times, it gives you the opportunity to discuss your project directly with colleagues and other professionals, answer questions, and get instant feedback. Posters are especially useful for highlighting practical improvements, patient outcomes, or innovative practices in healthcare settings, so they lend themselves well to audits and service evaluations. A poster can be erroneously seen as an easier option to present, but it can actually be harder than you anticipate to get a poster right – getting the balance right between too much and too little information is key, and you should look at examples of posters in your clinical area and online posters to gauge what will be right for your target audience. An example of a conference poster is shown in Figure 7.1.

However, an oral presentation is perhaps seen as the more standard way of conveying the findings of your project to your target audience. Unlike posters, oral presentations usually involve a short talk, often supported by slides, and allow for structured discussion and questions from your audience. You are able to explain your project, highlight the key findings, explain the significance for healthcare practice, and answer questions in real time. Oral presentations are valuable for building your confidence, networking with other professionals, and raising the visibility of your project, so are a good option for any small-scale research project.

So, you should plan for an oral or poster presentation at a conference. Your place of work might organise conference days for staff or your university might have a student showcase conference, or an international nurses day conference or similar, all of which are great options for presenting your project, especially to a local, interested audience.

Professional/practice-based dissemination

Workplace or community reports

It will also be useful at a local level to share your findings with the organisation or community in which you conducted your research. This is particularly relevant for audits and service evaluations but also valuable for someone doing a small-scale research project. Workplace or

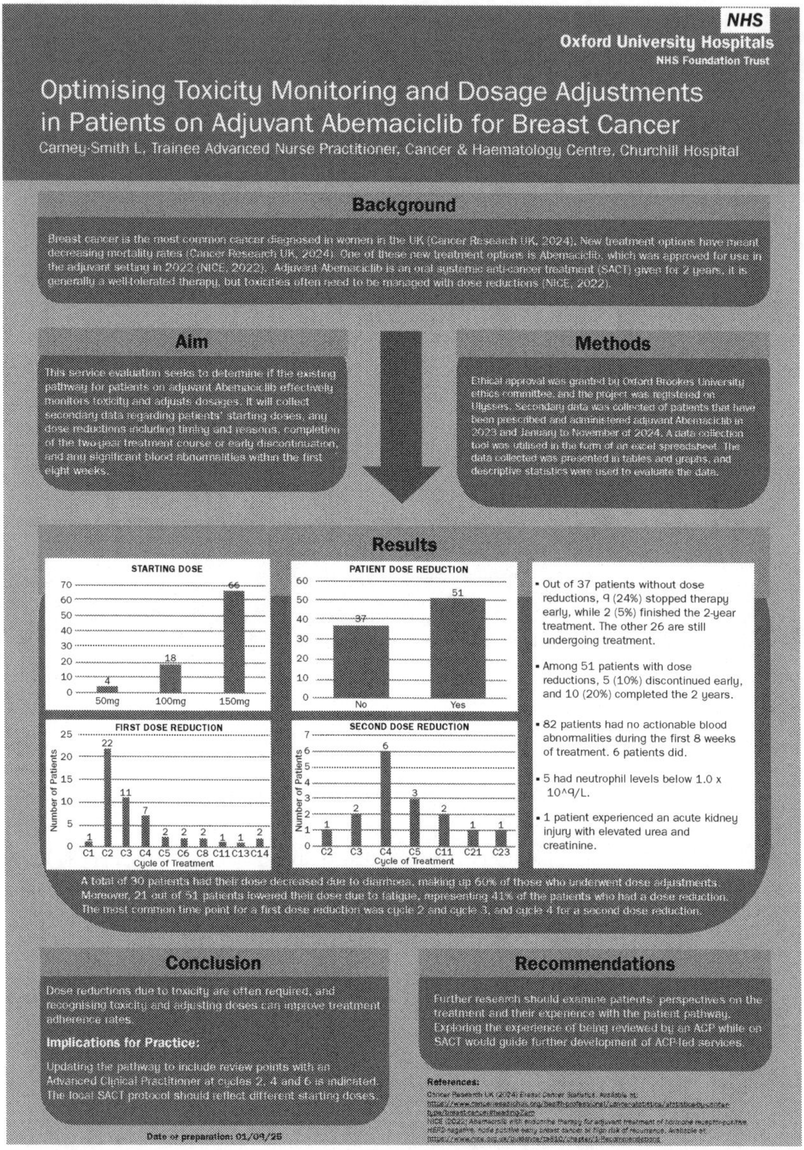

Figure 7.1 A conference poster from a clinical practitioner project.

community reports are a practical way to share the results of a health-care research project, indeed your participants may feel very invested in your project and keen to know what the results are. Also, it is good ethical research practice to offer your respondents an opportunity to review your results.

These reports need to be written in clear, accessible language suitable for colleagues, staff, managers or community groups rather than an academic audience. Within such a report you can highlight key findings, explain their relevance to practice, and offer recommendations for change or improvement. This allows you to use evidence-based practice to demonstrate real-world impact as well as working towards better outcomes for patients. An example is an openly available web page created by a doctoral student to keep participants, colleagues and the wider public informed of the progress of their project (see https://sites.google.com/brookes.ac.uk/liz-jestico-phd-study/home). This website is an example of good practice in using a contemporary method of communicating about a project and its findings (Jestico et al. 2023).

Workshops or presentations

Similar to conference presentations, these give you an opportunity to present to practitioners, service providers or local stakeholders who might benefit from your results. It's also useful to look out for local bulletins for your speciality, or regional or national speciality meetings at which you can present your findings, whilst acknowledging that they might not just be relevant to your local unit but may be of interest to others.

Birch (2024) was asked to present the findings of a service evaluation to the local governance team, and they reflect on this in Box 7.1.

Box 7.1: Reflections on a service evaluation

It was always deeply important to me that the topic for my dissertation be an area that I felt strongly about. I hoped to carry out primary research that may be of real use and relevance to current practice. I look forward to presenting my findings at the Quality Assurance Audit meeting. It will be a wonderful opportunity through which some of my recommendations may be taken into consideration. I have thoroughly enjoyed the dissertation process, and I am also excited for the possibility of prospective projects that have come to light as a result of the findings of this dissertation.

Similarly, Carney-Smith (2025) was able to reflect on the positive outcomes of their master's-level service evaluation and how it led to a direct change in the way breast cancer care is provided by advanced nurse practitioners in their Trust (see Box 7.2).

Box 7.2: Reflections of an advanced nurse practitioner on service evaluation

The service evaluation titled 'Optimising toxicity assessment and dosage adjustments in patients on adjuvant abemaciclib for breast cancer' was very well received by colleagues and the Trust. As this is a new treatment recently approved by NICE, there is often a need to learn and adapt as we go, so evaluating at this stage was extremely valuable. The proactive approach was appreciated, particularly as the recommended changes were implemented without requiring additional funding by reallocating resources within the team. These changes have positively impacted the patient pathway by improving prompt recognition of toxicities and timely dosage adjustments.

For my own practice, the evaluation has made a significant difference. I have established a dedicated clinic led by an advanced nurse practitioner to care for patients on this treatment, and I plan to review its impact in one year. Completing this evaluation has given me great confidence and strengthened my commitment to embedding research into everyday practice as an advanced nurse practitioner.

Public engagement

Public engagement is a relatively new concept whereby researchers endeavour to reach out to the public to share their findings. In many universities, there are specific roles devoted to this task as the need to engage the public in the work of local universities is a way of demonstrating accountability, improving the quality and relevance of research, and strengthening institutional ties with the community. You might decide that a very accessible way to share your findings would be via a podcast, blog or online article. These tend to be short pieces so are not onerous in their commitment to craft them, but you do need to make them in an accessible format for your audience.

Figure 7.2 is an example of a post in a departmental newsletter explaining about a project and providing a link to the resultant podcast. The university podcast series it is from is 'Oxford Brookes Unscripted', used to informally share, discuss and contemplate research with the wider community. It is open access and available from major podcast hosting services or via the following link: https://radar.brookes.ac.uk/radar/items/c8609d08-f0eb-4254-a662-b41564b36170/1/.

Of course, social media is an easy, interactive way of disseminating your results, whether that be on LinkedIn, X (formerly Twitter), a thread or any other social media platform. Social media allows for bite-size chunks of information to be posted, so it might be that you'd need to do several posts or more likely signpost within your thread to the other ways you are disseminating your results (e.g. poster at a conference, publication). You will also need to plan a punchy 'take home message' from your post and maybe also consider something visual or a graphic as a key takeaway or to make the reader want to know more. Providing links to more information or creating hashtags is ideal to enable your research to be discovered, categorised and engaged with. Think of hashtags as topic labels that help your audience find you. Social media has the potential for a much wider reach and consequently collaborations and the building up of your professional network. So, it can be very beneficial, but you do need to act ethically and responsibly – no one is there to moderate what you upload, there is no peer review, and you will need to stand by what you have posted in years to come, so take time to ponder and consider what you post before you upload to the internet.

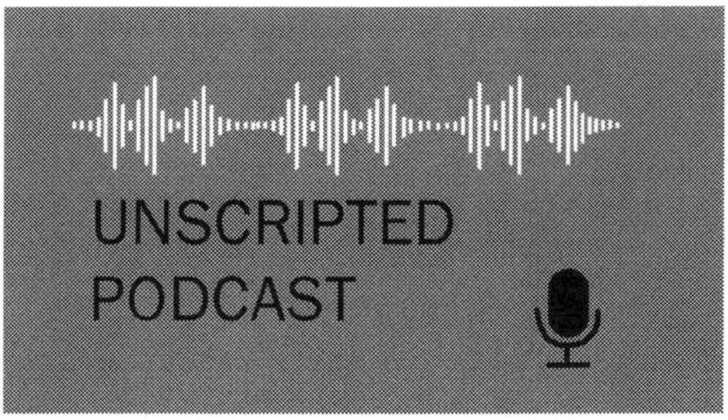

Dr. Marion Waite, Professor Vanessa Heaslip, and Dr. Louise Stayt to explore the ethical and human dimensions of digital nursing. At the frontline of digital transformation, our guests reflect on identity, inclusion, and the evolving role of technology in care. From the impact of social media on professional identity to the risks of excluding vulnerable populations in digital service design, the episode unpacks how nurses navigate a rapidly changing healthcare landscape. Drawing on their co-authored book chapter, the team calls for more inclusive, ethical, and user-informed approches to digital innovation. Their message is clear: one size does not fit all, and nurses must have a seat at the digital table.

Figure 7.2 Newsletter with a link to a podcast.

Other ideas

Collaborate with colleagues or your supervisor to take your small-scale research project forward – what you have done will lead to new ideas and enthusiasm to find out more; indeed, you might feel ready to embark on doctoral study, perhaps using your own findings as the foundations for your doctoral research question. Being on the lookout for funding calls such as those offered via the NIHR (https://www.nihr.ac.uk/funding-opportunities), is an excellent way to further your project or to prove to the selection panel that you have research experience. Or perhaps engaging in the research has led you to want to teach in a higher education institution, as research should always be embedded within the curriculum, and your experience may lead to opportunities to share your learning with others or even take on roles such as a teaching fellow or a visiting lecturer.

Key points

- Dissemination of your results is important as it reflects and honours the efforts of yourself, your participants and your supervisor.
- Do not consider the final write up of the project as the end point; there is more you can do to maximise the output from your work.
- Publication helps to give both you and your project a 'voice'.
- You will likely need to report audit results to a board or management team to determine if standards are being adhered to or not.
- You should think carefully about what methods of dissemination are best suited to your audience and to your project.
- Not all feedback is positively received and you should plan for this.

Concluding remarks

In this book we have outlined what you need to consider when undertaking an empirical study, be that an audit, service evaluation or small-scale research project. Despite their differences, they often use the same methods. So, there are more similarities than differences between them and all are great learning opportunities, even if your particular project does not warrant the official label of 'research'.

All projects benefit from a short literature review in order to ascertain any gap in the knowledge base, whether it is a research project, an audit or an evaluation of a current service. The degree to which you do this will depend on the requirements of your academic institution.

If you are undertaking a small-scale research project, when time is of the essence, we recommend that you focus on your research question rather than the wider philosophical debate. For this reason, any discussion of paradigms and methodologies will be secondary to the discussion and justification of the methods you use. However, it is necessary for the paradigm and methodology to be in alignment even if these are not explicitly described.

We strongly recommend you err on the side of pragmatism when choosing your methods. Be sensible about the scope of your project, as attention to detail will take up most of your time. Remember, you have to work within the time frame and resources available to you.

Once you have completed your project, and you have achieved what you set out to do, consider the wider impact your work might have. This is obviously an extra step but it will enable you to consolidate what you have achieved, take ownership of it and use it to influence others – be this with a publication, conference presentation or social media post.

Good luck!
Ginny and Kathleen and Helen

Postscript: reporting guidelines for writing up your small-scale research project

In the event you decide to publish your findings, there are reporting guidelines you will need to follow, which you can access via the EQUATOR network (www.equator-network.org). These are discussed by Aveyard et al. (2023a). Following the appropriate reporting guidelines is an expectation of most academic journals, whose purpose is to ensure the accurate reporting of research. Adherence to the guidelines ensures that all the necessary information about a study is documented and that key facts are not left unsaid/unreported. If you plan to publish your project, familiarise yourself with the EQUATOR network website and try to identify an appropriate set of guidelines – for example, ENTREQ (Enhancing Transparency in Reporting the Synthesis of Qualitative Research), to be followed for the reporting of the synthesis of qualitative research, or COREQ (Consolidated Criteria for Reporting Qualitative Research), a 32-item checklist for interviews and focus groups.

There are no reporting guidelines for undertaking a small-scale research project for an academic award, such as those outlined in this book. In view of this, we list our own guidelines below. These do not supersede the guidelines of your sponsoring institution but instead are a guide to what, in our view, are the necessary components that you need to include for a small-scale research project (e.g. a master's dissertation).

Table C1 Reporting guidelines for small-scale research projects

Section (and suggested percentage of your dissertation) – dependent on the requirements of your academic institution and personal judgement	**What to include**	**Further information**
Introduction and Background (10%) (including clear justification for your research question) You will usually include both an Introduction (explaining the problem) and Background (further supporting evidence) but ensure the Introduction is relatively short and, at the end of the Background section, you state your research question	The Introduction and Background should reflect the broader picture and incorporate key dates and events. Start with a critical reflection on practice and what led you to settle on your research question	For audits and service evaluations, the term 'research study' is commonly applied, even if they generally fall outside the remit of research. These projects fall within quality improvement (rather than research)
Literature Review (10–20%)	This should be a distinct section, separate from the Introduction and Background. Include a focused question – which might be different from your overall research question. You may or may not choose to use a tool such as PICO to develop your question	For research projects, the aim of the Literature Review is to provide a summary of evidence highlighting the gap in the knowledge base. For a service evaluation or audit, the literature review should justify your rationale for choosing that particular service

(*continued*)

Methods (10–20%)	You need to provide a step-by-step outline of your method. Who made up your sample? Where were they located? How did you recruit them? Was this successful? How did you collect data? Was this successful? How did you record the data? How did you analyse the data?	Focus on methods rather than paradigms or methodology. Reference primary sources whose methods you followed. Refer to projects that have used a similar method here
Findings/Results (25%)	Clear documentation of findings. Be bold but ensure a clear representation of the findings	Make sure you answer the research question, aims and objectives!
Discussion (20%)	Start with a brief summary of your aim and findings/results but ensure this is not a repeat of the previous section. Make reference to other research, theory or policy	Do *not* present any data from your project in this section. You need instead to discuss the wider implications of your findings/results
Conclusion and Limitations (2%)	This should a very succinct summary of your entire project. Be honest about any limitations but also upbeat about what you have achieved	Limitations will almost always include reference to your project being small scale in nature
Recommendations and Implications for Practice (3%)	Ensure these are based on the outcome of your project	Avoid only suggesting 'further research' – although this might be one of your recommendations

References

Abel, Z. (2023) *How do 'RAID' huddles impact on the recognition and escalation of clinically deteriorating adults on acute hospital inpatient wards*, unpublished MSc dissertation, Oxford Brookes University.

Arifin, S.R.B.M., Cheyne, H., Maxwell, M. and Yousuf, A. (2021) The Malaysian women's experience of care and management of postnatal depression, *Clinical Practice and Epidemiology in Mental Health*, 17: 10 [https://doi.org/10.2174/1745017902117010010].

Aveyard, H. (2023) *Doing a Literature Review in Health and Social Care: A Practical Guide*, 5th edition. London: Open University Press.

Aveyard, H. and Bradbury-Jones, C. (2019) An analysis of current practices in undertaking literature reviews in nursing: findings from a focused mapping review and synthesis, *BMC Medical Research Methodology*, 19 (1): 105 [https://doi.org/10.1186/s12874-019-0751-7].

Aveyard, H., Greenway, K. and Parsons, L. (2023b) *A Beginner's Guide to Evidence-based Practice in Health and Social Care*, 4th edition. London: Open University Press.

Aveyard, H., Payne, S. and Preston, N. (2026) *A Post-graduate's Guide to Writing a Literature Review in Health and Social Care*, 3rd edition. London: Open University Press.

Aveyard, H., Preston, N. and Farquhar, M. (2025) *How to Read and Critique Research: A Guide for Nursing and Healthcare Students*. London: Sage.

Aveyard, H., Bradbury-Jones, C., Ring, N. and Flemming, K. (2023a) Which reporting guideline should I use and why?, *Journal of Clinical Nursing*, 32 (9/10): e15–e16 [https://doi.org/10.1111/jocn.16548].

Aveyard, H., Kolawole, A., Gurung, P., Cridland, E. and Kozlowska, O. (2022) Informed consent prior to nursing care: nurses' use of information, *Nursing Ethics*, 29 (5): 1244–1252 [https://doi.org/10.1177/09697330221095148].

Barbour, R. (2014) Quality of data analysis, in U. Flick, K. Metzler and W. Scott (eds.) *The SAGE Handbook of Qualitative Data Analysis*, pp. 496–509. London: Sage.

Beauchamp, T.L. and Childress, J.F. (1994) *Principles of Biomedical Ethics*, 4th edition. Oxford: Oxford University Press.

Bell, J., Waters, S. and Johnson, H. (2024) *Doing Your Research Project: A Guide for First-time Researchers*, 8th edition. London: Open University Press.

Belmont Report (1979) *Ethical Principles and Guidelines for the Protection of Human Subjects of Research* (The Belmont Report). Department of Health, Education, and Welfare [https://www.paho.org/sites/default/files/2025-08/belmont-report.pdf].

Birch, I. (2024) *A mixed-methods service evaluation of a 'rainbow clinic'*, unpublished MSc dissertation, Oxford Brookes University.

Blaxter, L., Hughes, C. and Tight, M. (2010) *How to Research*, 4th edition. Maidenhead: Open University Press.

Bothra, M., Nair, B. and Nair, S. (2025) Impact of a focused thesis writing workshop on knowledge and confidence of medical postgraduate students: a cross-sectional study, *Journal of the Association of Physicians of India*, 73 (10): 20–23.

Bowers, D. (2020) *Medical Statistics from Scratch: An Introduction for Health Professionals*, 4th edition. Hoboken, NJ: Wiley Blackwell.

Boynton, P. (2017) *The Research Companion: A Practical Guide for Those in the Social Sciences, Health and Development*, 2nd edition. London: Routledge.

Braun, V. and Clarke, V. (2022) *Thematic Analysis: A Practical Guide*. London: Sage.

Brookfield, S. (1993) On impostorship, cultural suicide, and other dangers: how nurses learn critical thinking, *Journal of Continuing Education in Nursing*, 24 (5): 197–205 [https://doi.org/10.3928/0022-0124-19930901-04].

Carney-Smith, L. (2025) *Optimizing toxicity monitoring and dosage adjustments in patients on adjuvant Abemaciclib for breast cancer*, unpublished MSc dissertation, Oxford Brookes University.

Carrera, J.S., Brown, P., Brody, J.G. and Morello-Frosch, R. (2018) Research altruism as motivation for participation in community-centered environmental health research, *Social Science and Medicine*, 196: 175–181 [https://doi.org/10.1016/j.socscimed.2017.11.028].

Cooke, A., Smith, D. and Booth, A. (2012) Beyond PICO: the SPIDER tool for qualitative evidence synthesis, *Qualitative Health Research*, 22 (10): 1435–1443 [https://doi.org/10.1177/1049732312452938].

Coughlan, C., Alexis, O., Matheson, L. and Watson, E. (2024) A systematic review of the follow-up priorities of colorectal cancer survivors, *Gastrointestinal Nursing*, 22 (9): 408–418 [https://doi.org/10.12968/gasn.2024.0024].

Creswell, J.W. (2022) *A Concise Introduction to Mixed Methods Research*, 2nd edition. London: Sage.

Creswell, J.W. and Creswell, J.D. (2023) *Research Design: Qualitative, Quantitative, and Mixed Methods Approaches*, 6th edition. Thousand Oaks, CA: Sage.

Creswell, J.W. and Plano Clark, V.L. (2018) *Designing and Conducting Mixed Methods Research*, 3rd edition. Thousand Oaks, CA: Sage.

Deming, W.E. (1986) *Out of the Crisis: Quality, Productivity and Competitive Position*. Cambridge: Cambridge University Press.

Denscombe, M. (2021) *The Good Research Guide: Research Methods for Small-scale Social Research Projects*, 7th edition. London: Open University Press.

Desborough, J., Bagheri, N., Banfield, M., Mills, J., Phillips, C. and Korda, R. (2016) The impact of general practice nursing care on patient satisfaction and enablement in Australia: a mixed methods study, *International Journal of Nursing Studies*, 64: 108–119 [https://doi.org/10.1016/j.ijnurstu.2016.10.004].

Dixon, B. (2006) Tragedy of the uncommon, *Current Biology*, 16 (8): R263–R264 [https://doi.org/10.1016/j.cub.2006.03.072].

Dodds, C., Keogh, P., Bourne, A., et al. (2021) The long and winding road: archiving and re-using qualitative data from 12 research projects spanning 16 years, *Sociological Research Online*, 26 (2): 269–287 [https://doi.org/10.1177/1360780420924044].

Elwick, H., Joseph, S., Becker, S. and Becker, F. (2010) *Manual for the Adult Carer Quality of Life Questionnaire (AC-QoL)*. London: Princess Royal Trust for Carers/University of Nottingham.

Ferreira, C. (2025) *A clinical audit on the management of acute otitis externa in an ear, nose and throat centre at a NHS Trust hospital in England*, unpublished MSc dissertation, Oxford Brookes University.

Fineout-Overholt, E. and Johnston, L. (2005) Teaching EBP: asking searchable, answerable clinical questions, *Worldviews on Evidence-based Nursing*, 2 (3): 157–160 [https://doi.org/10.1111/j.1741-6787.2005.00032.x].

Forde-Johnston, C. (2025) *An exploration of nurse-patient interactions in acute hospital settings when Electronic Patient Record (EPR) systems are used*, PhD thesis, Oxford Brookes University.

Gale, N.K., Heath, G., Cameron, E., Rashid, S. and Redwood, S. (2013) Using the framework method for the analysis of qualitative data in multidisciplinary health research, *BMC Medical Research Methodology*, 13: 117 [https://doi.org/10.1186/1471-2288-13-117].

George, T. and Aveyard, H. (2020) Improving access to primary care services for those on low income: voluntary advocacy, *British Journal of Community Nursing*, 25 (4): 162–166 [https://doi.org/10.12968/bjcn.2020.25.4.162].

Goffman, E. (1961) *Asylums: Essays on the Social Situation of Mental Patients and Other Inmates*. Garden City, NY: Anchor Books.

Grazioli, V.S., Graells, M., Schmutz, E., et al. (2024) Developing a capacity-building intervention for healthcare workers to improve communication skills and awareness of hard of hearing and D/deaf patients: results from a participatory action research study, *BMC Health Services Research*, 24: 301 [https://doi.org/10.1186/s12913-024-10574-3].

Guillermo-Scott, V. (2025) *A service evaluation to explore to what extent community hospital clinical healthcare teams perceive the care and rehabilitation delivered as person-centred*, unpublished MSc dissertation, Oxford Brookes University.

Harris, M. and Taylor, G. (2021) *Medical Statistics Made Easy 4*. Banbury: Scion Publishing.

Hartland, J. and Larkai, E. (2020) Decolonising medical education and exploring White fragility, *BJGP Open* 4 (5) [https://doi.org/10.3399/BJGPO.2020.0147].

Heale, R. and Twycross, A. (2015) Validity and reliability in quantitative studies, *Evidence Based Nursing*, 18 (3): 66–67 [https://doi.org/10.1136/eb-2015-102129].

Higgins, J., Thomas, J., Chandler, J., et al. (eds.) (2024) *Cochrane Handbook for Systematic Reviews of Interventions*, 2nd edition. Oxford: Wiley Blackwell.

Holland, K. and Watson, R. (2021) *Writing for Publication in Nursing and Healthcare: Getting it Right*. Hoboken, NJ: Wiley.

Imms, B. (2025) *A service evaluation of a nurse led, fast track Ventricular Tachycardia Clinic*, unpublished MSc dissertation, Oxford Brookes University.

Jestico, E.C.L., Schutz, S.E., Finlay, T.M.D., et al. (2023) How 'significant others' may support parents with decision-making about their child's cancer care: an integrative literature review, *Journal of Clinical Nursing*, 32 (9/10): 1821–1840 [https://doi.org/10.1111/jocn.16220].

Johns Hopkins University (2025) *Clinical research: What is it?* [https://www.hopkinsmedicine.org/research/understanding-clinical-trials/clinical-research-what-is-it].

Jones, K., Wilson-Keates, B. and Melrose, S. (2024) Using social media to recruit research participants: a literature review, *Nurse Researcher*, 32 (1): 28–34 [https://doi.org/10.7748/nr.2023.e1859].

Jones, M. and Rattray, J. (2015) Questionnaire design, in K. Gerrish and J. Lathlean (eds.) *The Research Process in Nursing*, pp. 413–425. Chichester: Wiley.

Kennedy, K.V., Tupetz, A., Boone, W., et al. (2025) Factors influencing the recruitment of diverse populations into pain research: findings from a qualitative study with underrepresented participants, *Pain*, 166 (10): e478–e486 [https://doi.org/10.1097/j.pain.0000000000003641].

Klompstra, L., Strömberg, A., Jaarsma, T. and Hendriks, J.M. (2025) Challenges and strategies for effective recruitment and retention of participants in clinical research studies, *European Journal of Cardiovascular Nursing*, 24 (5): 808–812 [https://doi.org/10.1093/eurjcn/zvae158].

Kuper, A., Lingard, L. and Levinson, W. (2008) Critically appraising qualitative research, *BMJ*, 337: a1035 [https://doi.org/10.1136/bmj.a1035].

Kvale, S. (1996) *InterViews: An Introduction to Qualitative Research Interviewing.* Thousand Oaks, CA: Sage.

Lascelles, K. (2024) *Entering and adjusting to a different and uncertain world: experiences and support needs of adult family members, partners and friends in England who care for an adult at risk of suicide*, DNurs thesis, Oxford Brookes University.

Liamputtong, P. (2011) *Focus Group Methodology: Principles and Practices.* London: Sage.

Limb, C., Fowler, A., Gundogan, B., Koshy, K. and Agha, R. (2017) How to conduct a clinical audit and quality improvement project, *IJS Oncology* 2 (6): e24 [https://doi.org/10.1097/IJ9.0000000000000024].

Lincoln, Y.S. and Guba, E.G. (1985) *Naturalistic Inquiry.* Beverly Hills, CA: Sage.

Maddison C. (2023) *The impact of clinical context on the practice assessor's perception of the student nurse's performance in placement: an exploratory narrative inquiry*, EdD thesis, Oxford Brookes University.

McCallum, K. (2022) *Death and dying in the emergency department: a phenomenological study of the experiences of family members and nursing staff*, PhD thesis, Oxford Brookes University.

Michalikova, A. (2026) *What are the viewpoints of healthcare professionals involved in diabetes management integrating mental health assessments into diabetes reviews*, unpublished MSc dissertation, Oxford Brookes University.

Milinic, T., Burdis, N., Gill, E., et al. (2025) Research coordinators' perspectives on recruitment of minoritized people with cystic fibrosis into clinical trials, *BMC Pulmonary Medicine*, 25: 325 [https://doi.org/10.1186/s12890-025-03707-9].

Mounce, G., Greenway, K., Brueton, V. and Aveyard, H. (2025) Approaches to concept clarification: issues for consideration, *Journal of Advanced Nursing*, 81 (5): 2243–2245 [https://doi.org/10.1111/jan.16553].

National Audit Office (2001) *A practical guide to sampling* [https://www.nao.org.uk/wp-content/uploads/2001/06/SamplingGuide.pdf].

National Institute for Health and Care Excellence (NICE) (2024) *Otitis externa: Scenario: Acute otitis externa* [https://cks.nice.org.uk/topics/otitis-externa/management/acute-otitis-externa/; last updated August 2025].

National Institute for Health and Care Research (NIHR) (2022) *Research Inclusion Strategy 2022–27* [https://www.nihr.ac.uk/about-us/who-we-are/research-inclusion/strategy-2022-27].

National Institute for Health and Care Research (NIHR) (2024a) *Our impact* [https://www.nihr.ac.uk/about-us/our-impact].

National Institute for Health and Care Research (NIHR) (2024b) *Embedding a research culture: From bench to bedside and beyond* [https://www.nihr.ac.uk/about-us/what-we-do/embedding-research-culture].

National Institute on Aging (2023) *What is clinical research?* [https://www.nia.nih.gov/health/clinical-trials-and-studies/what-are-clinical-trials-and-studies#what-is-clinical-research].

NHS Health Research Authority (HRA) (2024) *People-centred clinical research* [https://www.hra.nhs.uk/planning-and-improving-research/best-practice/people-centred-clinical-research/].

NHS Health Research Authority (HRA) (2025) *UK Policy Framework for Health and Social Care Research, version 3.3* [https://www.hra.nhs.uk/planning-and-improving-research/policies-standards-legislation/uk-policy-framework-health-social-care-research/].

O'Shea, E., Timmons, S. and Irving, K. (2025) Meaningful inclusion of people with dementia in interview research: adopting the 'intentional stance', *Frontiers in Dementia*, 4: 1596393 [https://doi.org/10.3389/frdem.2025.1596393].

Okiki, C., Giusmin, G. and Hunter, L. (2023) 'Only for the white': A qualitative exploration of the lived experiences of Black, Asian and Minority Ethnic midwifery students, *Nurse Education Today*, 131: 105982 [https://doi.org/10.1016/j.nedt.2023.105982].

Oozageer Gunowa, N., Hutchinson, M., Brooke, J., Aveyard, H. and Jackson, D. (2021) Pressure injuries and skin tone diversity in undergraduate nurse education: qualitative perspectives from a mixed methods study, *Journal of Advanced Nursing*, 77 (11): 4511–4524 [https://doi.org/10.1111/jan.14965].

Oudat, Q. and Bakas, T. (2023) Merits and pitfalls of social media as a platform for recruitment of study participants, *Journal of Medical Internet Research*, 25: e47705 [https://doi.org/10.2196/47705].

Page, M.J., McKenzie, J.E., Bossuyt, P.M., et al. (2021) The PRISMA 2020 statement: an updated guideline for reporting systematic reviews, *BMJ*, 372: n71 [https://doi.org/10.1136/bmj.n71].

Patino, C.M. and Ferreira, J.C. (2018) Inclusion and exclusion criteria in research studies: definitions and why they matter, *Jornal Brasileiro de Pneumologia*, 44 (2): 84 [https://doi.org/10.1590/S1806-37562018000000088].

Patten, M.L. (2016) *Questionnaire Research: A Practical Guide*, 4th edition. London: Routledge.

Peat, J.K. (2001) Analysing the data, in W. Xuan, K. Williams and J.K. Peat (eds.) *Health Science Research: A Handbook of Quantitative Methods*. London: Routledge.

Pugh, K. (2023) *A service evaluation to explore the process of beginning to provide antenatal care to pregnant women sekking asylum*, unpublished MSc dissertation, Oxford Brookes University.

Richardson, W.S. and Murphy, A.L. (1998) Ask, and ye shall retrieve, *Evidence Based Medicine*, 3 (4): 100 [https://doi.org/10.1136/ebm.1998.3.100].

Robson, C. (2024) *Real World Research: A Resource for Users of Social Research Methods in Applied Settings*. Chichester: Wiley.

Scocco, P., Castriotta, C., Toffol, E. and Preti, A. (2012) Stigma of Suicide Attempt (STOSA) scale and Stigma of Suicide and Suicide Survivor (STO-SASS) scale: two new assessment tools, *Psychiatry Research*, 200 (2/3): 872–878 [https://doi.org/10.1016/j.psychres.2012.06.033].

Senek, M., Robertson, S., Ryan, T., et al. (2020) The association between care left undone and temporary nursing staff ratios in acute settings: a cross-sectional survey of registered nurses, *BMC Health Services Research*, 20: 637 [https://doi.org/10.1186/s12913-020-05493-y].

Sollaci, L.B. and Pereira, M.G. (2004) The introduction, methods, results, and discussion (IMRAD) structure: a fifty-year survey, *Journal of the Medical Library Association*, 92 (3): 364–367.

Stewart, A. (2020) *An exploration of how a local population access health care services in rural India*, unpublished MSc dissertation, Oxford Brookes University.

Suhonen, R. (2014) Academic writing for publication – how to start and proceed?, *Scandinavian Journal of Caring Sciences*, 28 (2): 213–214 [https://doi.org/10.1111/scs.12142].

Thomas G. (2023) *How to Do Your Research Project: A Guide for Students.* London: Sage.

Toepoel, V. (2016) *Doing Surveys Online.* London: Sage.

Wasti, S.P., Simkhada, P., van Teijlingen, E.R., Sathian, B. and Banerjee, I. (2022) The growing importance of mixed-methods research in health, *Nepal Journal of Epidemiology*, 12 (1): 1175–1178 [https://doi.org/10.3126/nje.v12i1.43633].

Watson, R. (2018) Starting the 'Discussion' section of a manuscript, *Nurse Author & Editor*, 28 (2): 1–5 [https://doi.org/10.1111/j.1750-4910.2018.tb00015.x].

Widdows, G. (2022) *A mexied methods service evaluation examining experiences and outcomes for women who chose intra-caesarean intra-uterine contraception*, unpublished MSc dissertation, Oxford Brookes University.

Winser, M. (2025) *Does the implementation of a digital triage process improve the appropriateness of referrals to an advanced care practitioner in primary care?*, unpublished MSc dissertation, Oxford Brookes University.

Wright, A.L., Willett, Y.J., Ferron, E.M., et al. (2024) Using social media to recruit participants in health care research: case study, *Journal of Medical Internet Research*, 26: e51751 [https://doi.org/10.2196/51751].

Yale, S., Brown, M. and Byrne, M. (2024) Using freedom of information requests to access novel data sources in health professions education research, *Postgraduate Medical Journal*, 101 (1195): 481–486 [https://doi.org/10.1093/postmj/qgae166].

Index

Page numbers with 't' are tables, with 'b' are boxes, and in italics are figures

Made in the USA
Coppell, TX
05 November 2026

11327619R00103